T0227237

Physical Medicine and Rehabilitation: An Update for Internists

Editor

DAVID A. LENROW

MEDICAL CLINICS
OF NORTH AMERICA

www.medical.theclinics.com

Consulting Editor
JACK ENDE

March 2020 • Volume 104 • Number 2

ELSEVIER

1600 John F. Kennedy Boulevard ● Suite 1800 ● Philadelphia, Pennsylvania, 19103-2899

http://www.theclinics.com

MEDICAL CLINICS OF NORTH AMERICA Volume 104, Number 2
March 2020 ISSN 0025-7125, ISBN-13: 978-0-323-72220-9

Editor: Katerina Heidhausen
Developmental Editor: Kristen Helm

Medical Clinics of North America (ISSN 0025-7125) is published bimonthly by Elsevier Inc., 360 Park Avenue South, New York, NY 10010-1710. Months of publication are January, March, May, July, September, and November. Business and editorial offices: 1600 John F. Kennedy Boulevard, Suite 1800, Philadelphia, PA 19103-2899. Periodicals postage paid at New York, NY, and additional mailing offices. Subscription prices are USD $295.00 per year (US individuals), $654.00 per year (US institutions), $100.00 per year (US Students), $353.00 per year (Canadian individuals), $850.00 per year (Canadian institutions), $200.00 per year for (foreign students), $100.00 per year for (Canadian students), $422.00 per year (foreign individuals), and $850.00 per year (foreign institutions). To receive student/resident rate, orders must be accompanied by name of affiliated institution, date of term, and the signature of program/residency coordinator on institution letterhead. Orders will be billed at individual rate until proof of status is received. Foreign air speed delivery is included in all Clinics' subscription prices. All prices are subject to change without notice. **POSTMASTER:** Send address changes to *Medical Clinics of North America*, Elsevier Health Sciences Division, Subscription Customer Service, 3251 Riverport Lane, Maryland Heights, Missouri 63043. **Customer Service: Telephone: 1-800-654-2452** (U.S. and Canada); **1-314-447-8871** (outside U.S. and Canada). **Fax: 314-447-8029. E-mail: journalscustomerserviceusa@elsevier.com** (for print support); **journalsonlinesupport-usa@elsevier.com** (for online support).

Reprints. For copies of 100 or more of articles in this publication, please contact the Commercial Reprints Department, Elsevier Inc., 360 Park Avenue South, New York, NY 10010-1710. Tel.: 212-633-3874; Fax: 212-633-3820; E-mail: reprints@elsevier.com.

Medical Clinics of North America is also published in Spanish by McGraw-Hill Interamericana Editores S. A., P.O. Box 5-237, 06500 Mexico, D.F., Mexico.

Medical Clinics of North America is covered in *MEDLINE/PubMed (Index Medicus), Current Contents, ASCA, Excerpta Medica, Science Citation Index,* and *ISI/BIOMED.*

PROGRAM OBJECTIVE
The goal of the *Medical Clinics of North America* is to keep practicing physicians up to date with current clinical practice by providing timely articles reviewing the state of the art in patient care.

TARGET AUDIENCE
All practicing physicians and other healthcare professionals.

LEARNING OBJECTIVES
Upon completion of this activity, participants will be able to:
1. Review the medical and rehabilitation management from acute diagnosis to chronic impairments of stroke, as well as moderate to severe Traumatic Brain Injury.
2. Discuss how exercise can maintain health and treat several disease processes, as well as provide effective long-term treatment.
3. Recognize treatment protocols utilized to help patients return to athletics and minimize future risk of injury.

ACCREDITATION
The Elsevier Office of Continuing Medical Education (EOCME) is accredited by the Accreditation Council for Continuing Medical Education (ACCME) to provide continuing medical education for physicians.

The EOCME designates this journal-based CME activity for a maximum of 11 *AMA PRA Category 1 Credit*(s)™. Physicians should claim only the credit commensurate with the extent of their participation in the activity.

All other healthcare professionals requesting continuing education credit for this enduring material will be issued a certificate of participation.

DISCLOSURE OF CONFLICTS OF INTEREST
The EOCME assesses conflict of interest with its instructors, faculty, planners, and other individuals who are in a position to control the content of CME activities. All relevant conflicts of interest that are identified are thoroughly vetted by EOCME for fair balance, scientific objectivity, and patient care recommendations. EOCME is committed to providing its learners with CME activities that promote improvements or quality in healthcare and not a specific proprietary business or a commercial interest.

The planning committee, staff, authors and editors listed below have identified no financial relationships or relationships to products or devices they or their spouse/life partner have with commercial interest related to the content of this CME activity:
Benjamin Abramoff, MD, MS; Kim Barker, MD; Franklin E. Caldera, DO, MBA; Allison Capizzi, MD; Sarah Eickmeyer, MD; Mark I. Ellen, MD; Jack Ende, MD, MACP; Katerina Heidhausen; Kristen Helm; M. Kristi Henzel, MD, PhD; Marilu Kelly, MSN, RN, CNE, CHCP; Cristina Kline-Quiroz, DO; Haewon Lee, MD; David A. Lenrow, MD, JD; Christina Lin, MD; Leroy R. Lindsay, MD; Robert Samuel Mayer, MD, MEHP; Amira Noles, MD; Phalgun Nori, MD; Michael W. O'Dell, MD; Binnan Ong, DO, MSBE; Adrian Popescu, MD; Keith M. Robinson, MD; Michael D. Stubblefield, MD; Jeyanthi Surendrakumar; Randel Swanson, DO, PhD; Diane A. Thompson, MD, MS; Monica Verduzco-Gutierrez, MD; Dominique Vinh, MD, MBA; James R. Wilson, DO; Jean Woo, MD.

UNAPPROVED/OFF-LABEL USE DISCLOSURE
The EOCME requires CME faculty to disclose to the participants;
1. When products or procedures being discussed are off-label, unlabelled, experimental, and/or investigational (not US Food and Drug Administration [FDA] approved); and
2. Any limitations on the information presented, such as data that are preliminary or that represent ongoing research, interim analyses, and/or unsupported opinions. Faculty may discuss information about pharmaceutical agents that is outside of FDA-approved labelling. This information is intended solely for CME and is not intended to promote off-label use of these medications. If you have any questions, contact the medical affairs department of the manufacturer for the most recent prescribing information.

TO ENROLL
To enroll in the *Medical Clinics of North America* Continuing Medical Education program, call customer service at 1-800-654-2452 or sign up online at http://www.theclinics.com/home/cme. The CME program is available to subscribers for an additional annual fee of USD $300.00.

METHOD OF PARTICIPATION

In order to claim credit, participants must complete the following;
1. Complete enrolment as indicated above.
2. Read the activity.
3. Complete the CME Test and Evaluation. Participants must achieve a score of 70% on the test. All CME Tests and Evaluations must be completed online.

CME INQUIRIES/SPECIAL NEEDS

For all CME inquiries or special needs, please contact elsevierCME@elsevier.com.

MEDICAL CLINICS OF NORTH AMERICA

SERIES OF RELATED INTEREST

Physical Medicine and Rehabilitation Clinics of North America
https://www.pmr.theclinics.com/
Primary Care: Clinics in Office Practice
https://www.primarycare.theclinics.com/

Contributors

CONSULTING EDITOR

JACK ENDE, MD, MACP
The Schaeffer Professor of Medicine, Department of Medicine, Perelman School of Medicine, University of Pennsylvania, Philadelphia, Pennsylvania

EDITOR

DAVID A. LENROW, MD, JD
Associate Professor, Department of Physical Medicine and Rehabilitation, University of Pennsylvania, Philadelphia, Pennsylvania

AUTHORS

BENJAMIN ABRAMOFF, MD, MS
Assistant Professor, Department of Physical Medicine and Rehabilitation, University of Pennsylvania, Philadelphia, Pennsylvania

KIM BARKER, MD
Associate Professor, Department of Physical Medicine and Rehabilitation, UT Southwestern Medical Center, Dallas, Texas

FRANKLIN E. CALDERA, DO, MBA
Associate Professor, Department of Physical Medicine and Rehabilitation, University of Pennsylvania, Philadelphia, Pennsylvania

ALLISON CAPIZZI, MD
Department of Physical Medicine and Rehabilitation, McGovern Medical School, The University of Texas Health Science Center at Houston, Houston, Texas

SARAH EICKMEYER, MD
Associate Professor, Department of Physical Medicine and Rehabilitation, University of Kansas Medical Center, Kansas City, Kansas

MARK I. ELLEN, MD
Birmingham, Alabama

M. KRISTI HENZEL, MD, PhD
Assistant Chief, Spinal Cord Injuries and Disorders Center, Louis Stokes Cleveland VA Medical Center, Assistant Professor, Department of Physical Medicine and Rehabilitation, Case Western Reserve University, MetroHealth System, Cleveland, Ohio

CRISTINA KLINE-QUIROZ, DO
Cancer Rehabilitation Medicine Fellow, MedStar Health/Georgetown, National Rehabilitation Hospital, Washington, DC

HAEWON LEE, MD
Clinical Assistant Professor, Physical Medicine and Rehabilitation, Department of Orthopedic Surgery, University of California, San Diego, San Diego, California

CHRISTINA LIN, MD
Senior Resident, Department of Physical Medicine and Rehabilitation, Johns Hopkins School of Medicine, Baltimore, Maryland

LEROY R. LINDSAY, MD
Department of Rehabilitation Medicine, Assistant Professor of Clinical Rehabilitation Medicine, Weill Cornell Medical College, New York, New York

ROBERT SAMUEL MAYER, MD, MEHP
Associate Professor, Department of Physical Medicine and Rehabilitation, Johns Hopkins School of Medicine, Baltimore, Maryland

AMIRA NOLES, MD
Chief Resident Physician, Department of Physical Medicine and Rehabilitation, Johns Hopkins School of Medicine, Baltimore, Maryland

PHALGUN NORI, MD
Clinical Assistant Professor, Department of Physical Medicine and Rehabilitation, Rutgers New Jersey Medical School, Clinical Chief, Kessler Institute for Rehabilitation, West Orange, New Jersey

MICHAEL W. O'DELL, MD
Department of Rehabilitation Medicine, Vice Chair and Professor of Clinical Rehabilitation Medicine, Weill Cornell Medical College, New York, New York

BINNAN ONG, DO, MSBE
Staff Physician, Spinal Cord Injuries and Disorders Center, Louis Stokes Cleveland VA Medical Center, Assistant Professor, Department of Physical Medicine and Rehabilitation, Case Western Reserve University, MetroHealth System, Cleveland, Ohio

ADRIAN POPESCU, MD
Assistant Professor, Department of Physical Medicine and Rehabilitation, Hospital of the University of Pennsylvania, Perelman School of Medicine, Philadelphia, Pennsylvania

KEITH M. ROBINSON, MD
Associate Professor, Department of Physical Medicine and Rehabilitation, Perelman School of Medicine, University of Pennsylvania, Corporal Michael J. Crescenz VA Medical Center, Philadelphia, Pennsylvania

MICHAEL D. STUBBLEFIELD, MD
Clinical Professor, Department of Physical Medicine and Rehabilitation, Rutgers New Jersey Medical School, National Medical Director for ReVital Cancer Rehabilitation, Select Medical, Medical Director for Cancer Rehabilitation, Kessler Institute for Rehabilitation, West Orange, New Jersey

RANDEL SWANSON, DO, PhD
Assistant Professor, Department of Physical Medicine and Rehabilitation, Perelman School of Medicine, University of Pennsylvania, Corporal Michael J. Crescenz VA Medical Center, Philadelphia, Pennsylvania

DIANE A. THOMPSON, MD, MS
Department of Rehabilitation Medicine, Assistant Professor of Clinical Rehabilitation Medicine, Columbia University Vagelos College of Physicians and Surgeons, Medical Director of the Inpatient Rehabilitation Unit, NewYork-Presbyterian Hospital, New York, New York

MONICA VERDUZCO-GUTIERREZ, MD
Associate Professor and Vice Chair of Quality, Compliance and Patient Safety, Department of Physical Medicine and Rehabilitation, McGovern Medical School, The University of Texas Health Science Center at Houston, Medical Director, Brain Injury and Stroke Programs, TIRR Memorial Hermann Hospital, Houston, Texas

DOMINIQUE VINH, MD, MBA
Assistant Professor, Department of Physical Medicine and Rehabilitation, Johns Hopkins School of Medicine, Baltimore, Maryland

JAMES R. WILSON, DO
Staff Physician, Spinal Cord Injuries and Disorders Center, Louis Stokes Cleveland VA Medical Center, Assistant Professor, Department of Physical Medicine and Rehabilitation, Case Western Reserve University, MetroHealth System, Cleveland, Ohio

JEAN WOO, MD
H. Ben Taub Department of Physical Medicine and Rehabilitation, Baylor College of Medicine, Houston, Texas

Contents

treatment. These impairments may include fatigue, pain, neuropathy, lymphedema, or radiation fibrosis syndrome and have the potential to deleteriously impact their function and quality of life. Cancer rehabilitation is a comprehensive resource that facilitates maximizing and maintaining cancer survivors' physical, social, psychological, and vocational functioning. This article covers the common functional impairments experienced by cancer survivors and the treatment strategies used in cancer rehabilitation. Application of these services can enhance the ongoing care for cancer survivors.

Cancer affects millions of individuals, and approximately half will develop functional impairments. Cancers that commonly, either from direct effects or from its treatments, result in functional impairments include breast, head and neck, brain, and spinal cord tumors. There is a plethora of potential impairments including pain, spasticity, dystonia, weakness, and neurogenic bowel or bladder. This article reviews the functional impairments frequently encountered in breast, head and neck, brain, and spinal cord tumors. The authors also discuss management and treatment options incorporated in comprehensive cancer rehabilitation to address these impairments to maximize and maintain function and quality of life.

Individuals with spinal cord injuries or disorders (SCI/D), whether of traumatic or nontraumatic cause, require multidisciplinary management by their care team to achieve optimal health outcomes. SCI/D is relatively rare in the general population and primary care providers (PCPs) may not have extensive experience managing people with these disorders. Spinal cord injuries, impair the body's autonomic and biomechanical performance by interrupting the communications to and from major bodily systems. This article provides a framework to help PCPs understand how these changes impact their patient's physiologic function and subsequent risks for health complications with guidance for initial treatment approaches.

Neck pain is the fourth leading cause of disability. Acute neck pain largely resolves within 2 months. History and physical examination play a key role in ruling out some of the more serious causes for neck pain. The evidence for pharmacologic interventions for acute and chronic musculoskeletal neck pain is limited. Lower back pain is the leading cause of disability and productivity loss. Consultation with a physical medicine and rehabilitation spine specialist within 48 hours for acute pain and within 10 days for all patients with lower back pain may significantly decrease rate of surgical interventions and increase patient satisfaction.

Foreword
Medical Care That Matters

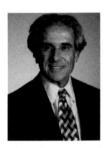

Jack Ende, MD, MACP
Consulting Editor

Medicine is a team sport. Internists, other primary care providers, subspecialists, radiologists, nurses, therapists, and so many others work together and, it is hoped, provide care that is as coordinated as it is comprehensive. But this care must also extend beyond the episode of the acute illness. Consider, for example, the patient in the hospital. Suppose the patient is ready for discharge. Then what happens? Ideally, the patient has improved and returns to his or her previous level of function. But we all know, for so many of our patients, including those with stroke, cancer, cardiopulmonary disease, neurologic disorders, and trauma, that may be the exception, not the rule.

Perhaps, then, the most important members of the team are our colleagues in Physical Medicine and Rehabilitation (PM&R). Their careers are devoted to enabling patients to regain function, or to adapt in the best way possible when function is lost. That is why, as the new Consulting Editor for the *Medical Clinics of North America*, I chose this update in PM&R as the topic of my first issue, and I am glad I did. Under the direction of Guest Editor, Dr David Lenrow, Associate Professor of PM&R at the Perelman School of Medicine at the University of Pennsylvania, this issue provides the latest evidence-based information spanning this very broad field from sports medicine to brain injury; from cardiopulmonary rehab to chronic care after hospitalization; and much more.

As physicians and other providers, we need to keep up with this important field. It is not possible to provide our patients with the best comprehensive and continuous care without addressing their rehabilitation needs. So, I encourage you to explore this issue

Med Clin N Am 104 (2020) xv–xvi
https://doi.org/10.1016/j.mcna.2019.11.005
0025-7125/20/© 2019 Published by Elsevier Inc.

medical.theclinics.com

and learn as much as you can. Medicine is, after all, a team sport, and our PM&R colleagues provide care over the long term when it may matter the most.

Jack Ende, MD, MACP
Department of Medicine
The Perelman School of Medicine at the University of Pennsylvania
5033 West Gates Pavilion
3400 Spruce Street
Philadelphia, PA 19104, USA

E-mail address:
jack.ende@uphs.upenn.edu

Preface

Physical Medicine and Rehabilitation: An Update for Internists

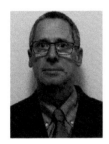

David A. Lenrow, MD, JD
Editor

Research and clinical care in the field of Physical Medicine and Rehabilitation (PM&R) have made tremendous advances since the field's early days of treatments predominantly with exercise and modalities. The focus of PM&R on patient function with a holistic approach has now spread to other specialties in medicine. The growth of the field has increased the presence of PM&R physicians in communities and hospitals providing treatment for patients with restrictions in function due to injury, illness, or disabling conditions. As society has become more accepting of persons with disabilities, maximizing function and independence has become more mainstream in health care.

The goal of this issue is to update the readership on advances in specific areas of PM&R so Internists will be aware of what the specialty has to offer patients and the treatment options available. Another important role in PM&R is the expertise in the determination of the appropriate level of post–acute care for patients who are hospitalized, be it outpatient rehabilitation services, home care, skilled nursing facilities, or acute hospital level rehabilitation.

Management of persons with chronic disabling conditions requires an understanding of the physiology and the specific needs of these patients. The issues are often quite different from patients without these conditions. An understanding of these issues allows for appropriately directed medical care for the specific needs of these patients. The articles in this issue review the unique needs of patients with some of the common chronic conditions that PM&R physicians care for and the specific approach to their care. Normal aging, pain, and injury are other topics covered with a focus on treatment and maximizing individual function.

Med Clin N Am 104 (2020) xvii–xviii
https://doi.org/10.1016/j.mcna.2019.11.006
0025-7125/20/© 2019 Published by Elsevier Inc.

I would like to thank all of the authors who graciously gave up their time to write the articles for this issue. The authors were selected from a variety of institutions for their expertise in the subject matter. These articles are a concise review of some of the pertinent issues and serve as a starting point to give the reader a broad understanding of the topics. The hope is that this will lead to increased interest and understanding and further investigation of topics of interest to assist in the care of patients.

Thank you to Elsevier for this opportunity to address their readership and review what PM&R has to offer for patient care. I hope that you are able to integrate some of the covered approaches to the care of your patients and, when appropriate, involve our specialty in the care of your patients.

David A. Lenrow, MD, JD
Department of Physical Medicine and Rehabilitation

University of Pennsylvania
Penn Medicine at Rittenhouse
1800 Lombard Street
Philadelphia, PA 19146, USA

E-mail address:
david.lenrow@uphs.upenn.edu

Therapeutic Exercise

Kim Barker, MD[a],*, Sarah Eickmeyer, MD[b]

KEYWORDS

- Exercise • Physical activity • Exercise prescription • Therapeutic exercise

KEY POINTS

- Physicians often overlook exercise as a treatment or prophylactic measure for many common diseases and ailments.
- Exercise can be used to treat comorbidities including obesity, cardiovascular disease, chronic obstructive pulmonary disease, diabetes mellitus, osteoporosis, osteoarthritis, cancer, and low back pain.
- Education on the general physical activity guidelines as well as easy exercise prescription methods can improve the ability of physicians to prescribe exercise as a therapeutic option.
- In addition, identifying barriers to compliance with exercise and ways to overcome these barriers is also necessary in order to use therapeutic exercise effectively.

INTRODUCTION

Modern American health care often emphasizes medications and procedures as treatment options. However, exercise is a valid, underused treatment option for many people. The benefits of exercise have been researched and documented by many groups, including the Centers for Disease Control and Prevention (CDC), the National Institutes of Health (NIH), the US Surgeon General, the American Heart Association (AHA), and the American College of Sports Medicine (ACSM).[1–3] These entities have released landmark publications on physical activity and health. Despite this, physical inactivity has been described as the greatest public health threat of the twenty-first century in the medical literature.[4] It is estimated that as low as 26% of men and 19% of women adhere to the guidelines. This low level of activity could have health and economic consequences costing as much as $100 billion.[5] This article reviews the physical activity guidelines for adult Americans, including aerobic, strengthening/resistance training, flexibility, and neuromotor training. This article also discusses how exercise can maintain health and treat several disease processes, as well as provide effective long-term treatment of these conditions.

a Department of Physical Medicine and Rehabilitation, UT Southwestern Medical Center, 5161 Harry Hines Boulevard, Dallas, TX 75390, USA; b Department of Physical Medicine and Rehabilitation, University of Kansas Medical Center, 3901 Rainbow Boulevard, Kansas City, KS 66160, USA
* Corresponding author.
E-mail address: kim.barker@utsouthwestern.edu

Med Clin N Am 104 (2020) 189–198
https://doi.org/10.1016/j.mcna.2019.10.003
0025-7125/20/© 2019 Elsevier Inc. All rights reserved.

medical.theclinics.com

EXERCISE GUIDELINES

The US Department of Health and Human Services (HHS) first published physical activity guidelines in 2008 and more recently in 2018. Inactivity is to be avoided and the recommendation is that adults exercise at least 2 d/wk. Ideally, the recommendation is to participate in at least 150 minutes of moderate-intensity or 75 minutes of vigorous-intensity aerobic exercise weekly. Individuals can also use a combination of both moderate-intensity and vigorous-intensity aerobic exercise. More gains can be expected if exercising more than 300 min/wk. The physical activity guidelines also emphasize resistance training, or strength training, twice a week (**Table 1**). Encouragement of balance activities using wobble boards or something as simple as walking backwards was also noted. Children and adolescents are recommended to participate in 60 minutes or more of aerobic activity daily, including bone and muscle strengthening activities. Some patient populations with various comorbidities are advised to check with a physician before starting an exercise program because of potential restrictions.[3,5]

EXERCISE PRESCRIPTION

Writing an exercise prescription can be difficult. The general exercise guidelines provide recommendations for a general target for many people, but many individuals benefit from specific directions. An exercise prescription should be designed to meet the specific needs of an individual person, geared to the person's comorbidities and age. Physiatrists (physician specialists in physical medicine and rehabilitation), in addition to physical therapists and athletic trainers, can be valuable resources in developing patients' programs. Exercise prescriptions involve careful screening, including history collection and physical examination, to determine the patient's capacity for physical activity, as well as a survey of goals and interests. Evidence shows that the benefits of regular physical activity are clear and far outweigh the inherent risk of adverse events.[6] Evaluating for issues such as cardiovascular, pulmonary, and metabolic health is an important part of an initial assessment.[7] Special consideration also needs to be placed on pain, which can serve as a barrier to exercise or lead to compensatory movement and ultimate failure.[8]

Patients should be counseled on appropriate timing to advance or reduce the exercise program. For people who have never exercised before, or if it has been a long time since they participated in regular exercise, the exercise prescription should be submaximal of the guidelines.[5] For instance, recommendations to start walking for just 5 minutes rather than the full 30 minutes may be all the person can tolerate. Gradual

Table 1	
United States Health and Human Services physical activity guidelines for adults	
Aerobic Activity	150–300 min/wk of moderate-intensity activity Or 75 min/wk of vigorous-intensity activity
Muscle Strengthening/ Resistance Exercises	Moderate or greater intensity involving all major muscle groups at least 2 d/wk

Data from U.S. Department of Health and Human Services. Physical Activity Guidelines for Americans, 2nd edition. Washington, DC: U.S. Department of Health and Human Services; 2018. Available at: https://health.gov/paguidelines/second-edition/pdf/Physical_Activity_Guidelines_2nd_edition.pdf. Accessed July 6 2019.

progression of activity is key. The persons performing the exercise should be focused on maintaining proper form and also on how their bodies feel while doing it. Insistence on good technique allows the patients to reach much higher levels of challenge and increase their strength and endurance gains with less risk of pain or injury. Finding the optimal dosage of load is also critical and considerations of alternatives such as high-intensity interval training (HIIT) or continuous aerobic training should be considered.[9] As the volume or quantity of the exercises builds, the patient may feel overwhelmed and at risk for abandoning the prescription. It can be helpful to have peer support or someone to check on the patient's progress intermittently. This support may improve motivation and compliance by allowing adjustments to be made accordingly in order to better achieve the desired outcomes.[7] In addition, a home exercise program should prepare the patients for their activities, fitness needs/goals, occupation, sport, or recreational activities. Many well-intended practitioners prescribe exercises that are appropriate and fit the suggestions discussed earlier, but do not assist the patient in returning to the desired job or activity because the home exercise program can only be performed in positions that are not supported by the environment. For example, supine exercises for low back pain given to a production line worker would not support a return to work activities. Other exercises can potentially put vulnerable areas under too much strain, such as using resistance bands or weights to try to strengthen a still painful rotator cuff injury.[7–9]

There are several methods of writing an exercise prescription. One of the easier methods is the FITT (frequency, intensity, time, and type) principle. The ACSM has expanded on this with the FITT-VP (frequency, intensity, time, type, volume, and progression) principle, which acknowledges the dynamic nature of an exercise prescription and allows for advancement. Each component of the exercise prescription mirrors a medication prescription and should include aerobic activity, resistance/strengthening, and stretching/flexibility training. Because the FITT-VP principle parallels the format of a typical medical prescription, it is fairly easy for most physicians to write.[7]

Greenman's[10] idea of exercise involves restoring length, strength, and control of muscle function as the process of treating muscular imbalances. A successful exercise program restores nervous system control of muscle function as much as possible. To achieve this, he prescribes the following sequence:

- Sensory motor balance training
- Stretching of short, tight, hypertonic muscle to symmetry
- Strengthening of inhibited weak muscles
- Restoration of symmetric movement patterns
- Aerobic conditioning

Another method of exercise prescription, outlined by McGill and colleagues,[8] takes on a 5-stage progression of training:

- Stage 1 involves detection and remedy of incorrect motor patterns.
- Stage 2 establishes stability of joints throughout the body via exercise and education, with a focus on spine stability.
- Stage 3 develops endurance and applies prior skills to daily activities.
- Stages 4 and 5 are for athletes and include training strength, speed, power, and agility.

Even with these exercise prescriptions and the HHS physical activity guidelines, there is still debate regarding the ideal volume and intensity of exercise in order to see therapeutic benefits. Current recommendations advise accumulation of moderate-intensity aerobic physical activity to attain a daily goal of around

30 minutes. However, additional data are available to show that shorter bouts of approximately 10 minutes each can be effective in attaining the same goal and suggest that the total volume of energy expended over a period of time is more important.[11] Large prospective studies of diverse populations show that a total energy expenditure of approximately 1000 kcal/wk of moderate-intensity physical activity is associated with lower rates of cardiovascular disease and premature mortality.[5] Significant risk reductions for cardiovascular disease have been shown to begin at volumes less than the recommended targets, and as low as one-half the recommended volume. Although measuring kilocalories is useful, perhaps a more practical measurement for aerobic activity is the metabolic equivalent (MET). METs measure the absolute intensity of aerobic activity, with 1 MET equivalent to the resting metabolic oxygen consumption rate of approximately 3.5 mL/kg/min. Significant health benefits emerge with a volume of 500 to 1000 MET minutes per week and this volume can be met by walking at 4.8 km/h (3.0 mile/h) on 3 d/wk for 50 minutes.[12]

A meta-analysis in 2016 quantified the dose-response association between physical activity and 5 chronic diseases (diabetes mellitus, ischemic heart disease, ischemic stroke, breast and colon cancer) and found that higher levels of total physical activity, compared with current minimums recommended, were associated with lower risk for all outcomes.[12] However, the dose-response relationship between volume and health benefits is curvilinear, with the greatest return on investment at lower levels of activity and decreasing return of health benefits at higher levels of activity.[13] It should also be kept in mind that although the recommendation to patients that some is good and more is better is well supported, there is also a role for smaller, well-spaced increments of exercise in order to reduce the incidence of adverse events and improve adherence.[13]

THERAPEUTIC EXERCISE FOR SPECIFIC PATIENT POPULATIONS

Although most of recommendations for exercise target general, healthy adults, evidence suggests that exercise can be particularly beneficial for patient populations with certain comorbidities. Therapeutic exercise can be used preventively or in conjunction as treatment of such diseases as obesity, heart disease, stroke, diabetes mellitus type 2, and certain cancers.

Obesity

The National Heart, Lung, and Blood Institute Obesity Education Initiative Expert Panel published a practical guide that recommends physical activity as an integral part of a comprehensive plan to treat obesity. Exercise increases a person's energy expenditure, which leads to weight loss as long as the energy expenditure is larger than the calories consumed. Thirty minutes of moderate activity is recommended for most, if not all, days of the week for obese patients. For this population, physical activity should be increased slowly in order to avoid musculoskeletal injury.[14] However, for substantial weight loss (>5% of a person's body weight), it is estimated that 300 minutes of moderate-intensity exercise per week is needed to meet this goal and maintain the weight loss.[5] A wide variety of activities may achieve this goal; walking, dancing, gardening, and sports are given as examples.[14] Resistance training is also helpful in reducing adipose tissue, including visceral adipose tissue.[15] Exercise in combination with diet produces the best outcomes with regard to improved lipid levels, fasting glucose level, and blood pressure.[16]

Cardiovascular Diseases

Physical activity's benefits on cardiorespiratory health are extensively well documented.[5] Heart disease and stroke risks can be dramatically decreased with exercise. Regular aerobic exercise is well known to decrease arterial stiffness, reduce blood pressure, increase high-density lipoprotein level, decrease low-density lipoprotein level, and decrease resting heart rate. Exercise is known to decrease all-cause mortality in patients with coronary artery disease.[5,17] However, what are often overlooked are the benefits of the addition of resistance training to aerobic exercise. Increasing skeletal muscle mass has similar effects as aerobic exercise and can complement the effects. Historically, several studies identified concerns that resistance training and strengthening exercises alone may increase arterial stiffness. However, some more recent studies have been inconclusive or contradictory, showing improvement in arterial stiffness.[15]

Results from HF-ACTION (Heart Failure: A Controlled Trial Investigating Outcomes of Exercise Training) suggest that exercise therapy reduces cardiac mortality and hospitalizations in patients with coronary heart disease and that exercise therapy may be safely conducted in certain heart failure populations.[18] A recent meta-analysis supports this evidence. It found reduction in the risk of rehospitalization caused by heart failure and improvements in health-related quality of life following exercise interventions.[19,20]

Chronic Obstructive Pulmonary Disease

With regard to pulmonary rehabilitation and exercise prescription in chronic obstructive pulmonary disease (COPD), a recent review found that, of the current 3 major guidelines, there was no optimal exercise prescription strategy established for COPD. The guidelines discussed were created by the American Association of Cardiovascular and Pulmonary Rehabilitation, the ACSM, and the American Thoracic Society/European Respiratory Society. The investigators advise that health care professionals should be familiar with all major, evidence-based pulmonary rehabilitation guidelines. The investigators also cite the core components of exercise training programs for COPD as endurance and resistance training.[21]

Diabetes Mellitus

The therapeutic effects of exercise on type 2 diabetes mellitus and its prevention is well known. The American Diabetic Association released a position statement on exercise in 2003, and again in 2006. It noted that physical activity should be promoted as a "vital component" of prevention and management of type 2 diabetes and, with the global epidemic of obesity, exercise should be a high priority.[22,23] It also noted that, despite concerns of hypoglycemia during exercise for people with type 1 diabetes, this population also benefits from exercise and that adjusting insulin and nutritional regimens (eg, supplementing with a carbohydrate) may be necessary to allow for activity.[22,23] A meta-analysis of 14 clinical trials in *JAMA* noted that exercise improved hemoglobin A1c levels significantly (from 7.65% to 8.31%, $P<.001$). However, improved glycemic control did not necessarily lead to a decrease in body mass in these trials. The most common type of exercise identified in the meta-analysis was moderately intense aerobic activity for 50 minutes, 3 times a week. Some studies also included resistance training in their exercises regimens, but not all. In addition, a few of the studies also included diet along with the exercise.[24] Exercise has also been shown to decrease the risk of developing many comorbid diseases, such as cardiovascular disease, hyperlipidemia, and hypertension.[22] In 2006, the American

Diabetes Association reached a consensus stance on exercise, stating that there is level A evidence for the therapeutic effect of aerobic and resistance exercise on glycemic control.[23]

Geriatrics

The benefits of exercise in the geriatric population are robust. This article narrows its focus on bone health, osteoarthritis, balance, and cognition.

In osteopenia and osteoporosis, there is strong evidence that bone health starts to decline with aging and as physical activity decreases.[5] To combat osteopenia and osteoporosis, impact and strengthening exercise that increase muscle mass have been shown to be preventive and therapeutic. This effect is particularly noted in postmenopausal women, in whom impact exercise therapeutically improves bone mineral density. One meta-analysis noted that a mix of loading exercise programs (eg, combining both low-impact loading, such as walking/stairs, along with higher-impact, such as jogging) increased bone mineral density better than high-impact alone.[25] Another review article also confirmed that combined exercise programs with mixed activities also increased quality of life by improving physical functioning outcomes (both short and long term), increased vitality, and also decreased pain domains.[26] Much of osteoporosis research focuses on women, but it has been proved in men that resistance training and impact-loading activities also improve bone health in middle-aged and older men.[27] HHS recommends 90 minutes of impact and strengthening exercises a week as treatment of declining bone health.[5]

With regard to osteoarthritis, exercise also has been proved to be helpful in improving functioning and decreasing pain in the short term. There is no specific type of exercise or amount. What is identified is that aerobic activity, strengthening (particularly in quadriceps and hamstring muscle groups), aquatic exercises, and tai chi have been shown to be beneficial for osteoarthritic pain. The major downside to exercise as treatment of osteoarthritis is compliance with this treatment regimen.[28] However, the long-term therapeutic benefits of exercise on osteoarthritis of the hip and knee are limited and not as encouraging. In a Cochrane Review focused specifically on osteoarthritis of the knee, the benefits of exercise seemed to last about 2 to 6 months.[29] Results in a different Cochrane Review of osteoarthritis of the hip were similar, showing pain improvement for 3 to 6 months.[30] This finding may be caused by the lack of adherence to the treatment plan over a prolonged period of time. Booster sessions to help improve compliance in the long term were shown to be beneficial for extended maintenance.[31]

Falls in the elderly are a major concern because hip fractures are a serious health condition and are associated with high rates of morbidity and mortality. In order to improve balance and reduce falls in the elderly, exercises that challenge balance are encouraged. Higher doses of exercise also seem to be beneficial. Interestingly, exercise regimens that primarily focused on walking were not found to be as beneficial. Based on 44 trials of various therapeutic exercise programs, an overall reduction of 17% was noted. This review also helps to show that exercises that challenge balance and may be typically avoided because of fear of falls do help to improve balance.[32] Other research has suggested that multicomponent exercise programs are successful at reducing falls. Programs that include strengthening, aerobic activity, balance training, and coordination at moderate intensity levels have improved balance.[5]

In recent years, there has been excitement about exercise's effect on cognition and potentially decreasing the risk of dementia. Some research shows that immediate results of exercise include improved anxiety and sleep. With long-term exercise, there is improvement in executive functioning, including the ability to plan and organize, attention, processing, and emotional control.[5] However, many studies have small enrollment and mixed results. In the few studies that do show benefit, it seems that tai chi improves attention and processing compared with no exercise.[33]

Cancer

The ACSM published guidelines for physical activity in cancer survivors in 2010 with general recommendations. The instruction is to avoid inactivity, and to continue exercise as soon and as often as possible.[34] Physical inactivity and obesity have been shown to increase people's risk of development and of recurrence of certain cancers, such as colon, breast, and endometrial.[35] For both aerobic and resistance exercises, the ACSM provided tumor-specific recommendations taking into account the pathophysiology and unique effects of specific cancer types (eg, risk of pathologic fractures from bone metastasis or the risk of lymphedema after mastectomy).[34] Resistance and strengthening have been shown to be safe in patients with postmastectomy lymphedema.[36] The ACSM recommends a "low and slow" approach, and no upper limit on the amount of resistance an individual is capable of progressing toward.[34] One randomized controlled trial noted that the combination of both moderate-intensity aerobic exercise and resistance training reduces the symptoms of chemotherapy-induced peripheral neuropathy when used during treatment.[37] Caution must be taken with overtraining in individuals with hematologic malignancies who received hematopoietic stem cell transplants, because of concern for adverse immune effects.[34]

Low Back Pain

Low back pain is one of the most common chief complaints seen in clinics in America, and therapeutic exercise is often underused. Although the literature is not as supportive in the role of treatment of acute back pain, exercise as treatment of chronic low back pain has been shown to decrease pain levels, improve functioning, and improve return-to-work outcomes.[35] Much attention has been directed recently at the importance of building core stability as a central focus of an exercise program. Because the core forms the link between the upper and lower body, the greater the stability of this part of the body, the more successful the movements and exercise program can be, with lower risk for certain injuries.[36–38] Additional evidence is available to support inclusion of proprioceptive-rich exercises as a part of the exercise program as well.[13,39]

BARRIERS TO COMPLIANCE

The major drawback to therapeutic exercise is compliance with the long-term treatment plan, which often contradicts a person's preference for a short-term, easy fix.[40] Patients note lack of time, lack of motivation, and poor ability to maintain adherence. There are tools to measure people's readiness to exercise more. The Physical Activity Readiness Questionnaire (PAR-Q) is a self-guided, 7-question tool that can be used as a screening instrument. Engagement and finding activities that the person will enjoy doing also help improve compliance with exercise.[7] For example, people who enjoy socializing with others may be more successful with consistent exercise when enrolled in group classes or participating in team sports rather than running on treadmills in their own homes alone. People who are motivated and engaged may be more willing to find the time to exercise, even if it means foregoing more enjoyable activities. Other barriers include pain (both premorbid as well as new onset caused by too rapid progression) and another medical condition that limits activity or the amount of activity done. Addressing these medical conditions, or finding an alternative exercise to accommodate, can be successful. For instance, a person with knee osteoarthritis that limits running may do well with swimming or water aerobics, in which the buoyancy of the water decreases the pain in the knees.[40,41] For those who cite time as a barrier, physicians can recommend using HIIT. A recent meta-analysis of HIIT for cardiometabolic health cited that, compared with moderate-intensity continuous aerobic training, HIIT may be more effective at increasing aerobic capacity and reducing risk factors associated with metabolic syndrome. Investigators of 1 study encourage clinicians to incorporate HIIT, performed 3 times a week for at least 12 weeks, into exercise programs for obese patients.[41] Another recent review of HIIT in patients with coronary heart disease found that the optimal protocol involved short interval durations (15 seconds) and maintaining close work/recovery ratios.[42]

DISCUSSION

Most exercise research is focused on outcomes for healthy adults. Although there are guidelines on volume, intensity, and frequency of exercise for healthy individuals, further investigation is needed into which exercises and what intensity and volumes are more beneficial for certain populations. Further investigation into these disease processes will better emphasize the preventive and curative effects of exercise. In addition, longitudinal studies to investigate how exercise affects people over their lifetimes will also be helpful in further defining exercise's role in maintaining health. Other directions include research and guidelines for people with physical disabilities, both congenital and acquired. The focus on acquired disability and aging will become more important in the United States as the population becomes older and faces new health challenges. With time, as research and the literature become more robust, it will become more evident that therapeutic exercise can be used in addition to medication and surgeries in the treatment of patients.

DISCLOSURE

The authors have nothing to disclose.

REFERENCES

1. Pate RR, Pratt M, Blair SN, et al. Physical activity and public health. A recommendation from the Centers for Disease and Prevention and the American College of Sports Medicine. JAMA 1995;273(5):402–7.
2. NIH Consensus Development Panel on Physical Activity and Cardiovascular Health. Physical activity and cardiovascular health. JAMA 1996;276(3):241–6.
3. U.S. Department of Health and Human Services. Physical activity and health: a report of the surgeon general. Atlanta (GA): U.S. Department of Health and Human Services, Public Health Service, CDC, National Center for Chronic Disease Prevention and Health Promotion; 1996. p. 278.
4. Blair SN. Physical inactivity: the biggest public health problem of the 21st century. Br J Sports Med 2009;43:1–2.
5. Azan A. Physical activity guidelines for Americans. 2nd edition. Washington, DC: U.S. Department of Health and Human Services; 2018. p. 78. Available at: https://health.gov/paguidelines/second-edition/pdf/Physical_Activity_Guidelines_2nd_edition.pdf. Accessed July 6, 2019.
6. Powell KE, Paluch AE, Blair SN. Physical activity for health: What kind? How much? How intense? On top of what? Annu Rev Public Health 2011;32:349–65.

7. Phillips EM, Kennedy MA. The exercise prescription: a tool to improve physical activity. PM R 2012;4:818–25.

8. McGill SM, Grenier S, Kavcic N, et al. Coordination of muscle activity to assure stability of the lumbar spine. J Electromyogr Kinesiol 2003;13:353–9.

9. McGill SM. Low back disorders, evidence-based prevention and rehabilitation. 2nd edition. Champaign (IL): Human Kinetics; 2007. p. 168.

10. Greenman PE. Principles of manual medicine. 2nd edition. Baltimore (MD): Williams & Wilkins; 1996. p. 456.

11. Garber CE, Blissmer B, Deschenes MR, et al. American College of Sports Medicine Position Stand: the quantity and quality of exercise for developing and maintaining cardiorespiratory, musculoskeletal, and neuromotor fitness in apparently healthy adults: guidance for prescribing exercise. Med Sci Sports Exerc 2011; 43(7):1334–59.

12. Buchner D. Physical activity. In: Goldman L, Schafer A, editors. Goldman's Cecil medicine, Vol. 2, 24th edition. Philadelphia: Saunders; 2016. p. 56–8.

13. Martinez-Amat A, Hita-Contreras F, Lomas-Vega R, et al. Effects of 12-week proprioception training program on postural stability, gait and balance in older adults: a controlled clinical trial. J Strength Cond Res 2013;27(8):2180–8.

14. Pi-Sunyer FX, Becker DM, Bouchard C, et al. National heart, lung and blood institute obesity education initiative expert panel. The practical guide: identification, evaluation, and treatment of overweight and obesity in adults. 2000. Available at: https://www.nhlbi.nih.gov/files/docs/guidelines/prctgd_c.pdf. Accessed July 6, 2019.

15. Braith R, Stewart K. Resistance exercise training: its role in the prevention of cardiovascular disease. Circulation 2006;113:2642–50.

16. Shaw K, Gennat H, O'Rourke P, et al. Exercise for overweight or obesity. Cochrane Database Syst Rev 2006;(4):CD003817.

17. Kodama S, Saito K, Tanaka S, et al. Cardiorespiratory fitness as a quantitative-predictor of all-cause mortality and cardiovascular events in healthy men and women; a meta-analysis. JAMA 2009;301(19):2024.

18. Forman D. Rehabilitation practice patterns for patients with heart failure: the United States perspective. Heart Fail Clin 2015;11(1):89–94.

19. Sagar VA, Davies EJ, Briscoe S, et al. Exercise-based rehabilitation for heart failure: systematic review and meta-analysis. Open Heart 2015;2:e000163.

20. Billinger S, Arena R, Bernhardt J, et al. Physical activity and exercise recommendations for stroke survivors: a statement for healthcare professionals from the American Heart Association/American Stroke Association. Stroke 2014;45(8): 2532–53.

21. Garvey C, Bayles M, Hamm L, et al. Pulmonary rehabilitation exercise prescription in chronic obstructive pulmonary disease: review of selected guidelines: an official statement from the American Association Of Cardiovascular And Pulmonary Rehabilitation. J Cardiopulm Rehabil Prev 2016;36(2):75–83.

22. American Diabetes Association. Physical activity/exercise and diabetes mellitus. Diabetes Care 2003;26(suppl1):s73–7.

23. Sigal RJ, Kenny GP, Wasserman DH, et al. Physical activity/exercise and type 2 diabetes: a consensus statement from the American Diabetes Association. Diabetes Care 2006;29(6):1433–8.

24. Boulé NG, Haddad E, Kenny GP, et al. Effects of exercise on glycemic control and body mass in type 2 diabetes mellitus: a meta-analysis of controlled clinical trials. JAMA 2001;286(10):1218–27.

25. Martyn-St James M, Carroll s. A meta-analysis of impact exercise on postmeno-pausal bone loss: the case for mixed loading exercise programmes. Br J Sports Med 2009;43:898–908.
26. Li WC, Chen Yc, Yang RS. Effects of exercise programmes on quality of life in osteoporotic and osteopenic postmenopausal women: a systematic review and meta-analysis. Clin Rehabil 2009;23(10):888–96.
27. Botam KA, van Uffelen JGZ, Taaffe DR. The effect of physical exercise on bone density in middle-aged and older men: a systematic review. Osteoporos Int 2013;24(11):2749–62.
28. Bennell KL, Hinman RS. A review of the clinical evidence for exercise in osteoar-thritis of the hip and knee. J Sci Med Sport 2011;14(1):4–9.
29. Fransen M, McConnell S, Harmer AR, et al. Exercise for osteoarthritis of the knee: a Cochrane systematic review. Br J Sports Med 2015;49:1554–7.
30. Fransen M, et al. Exercise for osteoarthritis of the hip. Cochrane Database Syst Rev 2014;4:1468–858.
31. Pisters MF, Veenhof C, van Meeteren NL, et al. Long-term effectiveness of exer-cise therapy in patients with osteoarthritis of the hip or knee: a systematic review. Arthritis Care Res 2007;57(7):1245–53.
32. Boyne P, Buhr S, Rockewell B. Predicting heart rate at the ventilatory threshold for aerobic exercise prescription in persons with chronic stroke. J Neurol Phys Ther 2015;39(4):233–40.
33. Uffelen JG, Chin A Paw MJ, Hopman-Rock M, et al. The effects of exercise on cognition in older adults with and without cognitive decline: a systematic review. Clin J Sports Med 2008;18(6):486–500.
34. Schmitz KH. American College of Sports Medicine roundtable on exercise guide-lines for cancer survivors. Med Sci Sports Exerc 2010;42(7):1409–26.
35. Eickmeyer s, Gamble GL, Shahpar S, et al. The role and efficacy of exercise in persons with cancer. PM R 2012;4(11):874–81.
36. McKenzie D, Kalda A. Effect of upper extremity exercise on secondary lymphe-dema in breast cancer patients: a pilot study. J Clin Oncol 2003;21(3):463–6.
37. Klickner I, Kamen C, Gewandter JS, et al. Effects of exercise during chemo-therapy on chemotherapy-induced peripheral neuropathy: a multi-center ran-domized controlled trial. Support Care Cancer 2018;26(40):1019–28.
38. Micheo W, Baerga L, Miranda G. Basic principles regarding strength, flexibility, and stability exercises. PM R 2012;4:805–11.
39. Willardson JM. Core stability training: application to sports conditioning pro-grams. J Strength Cond Res 2007;21(3):979–85.
40. Hoffman MD, Kraemer WJ, Judelson DA. Therapeutic exercise. In: Frontera W, Delisa J, Gans J, et al, editors. Delisa's physical medicine and rehabilitation. 5th edition. Philadelphia: Wolters Kluwer; 2010. p. 1634–62.
41. Batacan R, Duncan M, Dalbo V, et al. Effects of high-intensity interval training on cardiometabolic health: a systematic review and meta-analysis of intervention studies. Br J Sports Med 2016. https://doi.org/10.1136/bjsports-2015- 095841. Available at: http://bjsm.bmj.com/. Accessed January 1, 2017.
42. Ribeiro P, Boidin M, Juneau M, et al. High-intensity interval training in patients with coronary heart disease: Prescription models and perspectives. Ann Phys Rehabil Med 2017;60(1):50–7.

Updated Approach to Stroke Rehabilitation

Leroy R. Lindsay, MD[a],*, Diane A. Thompson, MD, MS[b], Michael W. O'Dell, MD[a]

KEYWORDS

- Stroke • Rehabilitation • Physiatry

KEY POINTS

- Physiatrists provide nonsurgical management of neurologic and orthopedic conditions, to improve mobility and function.
- Prevention, early recognition, and early intervention will likely limit the severity and cost of these post stroke conditions.
- Multidisciplinary rehabilitation teams create stroke rehabilitation programs that aim to improve the function and quality of life of stroke survivors.

PHYSIATRY AND COMMON SETTINGS FOR STROKE REHABILITATION

Stroke is now the leading cause of serious long-term disability in individuals older than 65. Each year more than 800,000 people in the United States will experience a stroke, with approximately 600,000 of these events being first events.[1] Although mortality has decreased in recent years, more than half will have significant deficits in mobility, cognition, and their ability to perform activities of daily living (ADLs).[1] Although great strides have been made in the realm of primary stroke prevention, management of modifiable risk factors, and initial stroke management, surviving the initial event is just the beginning of the journey. The incidence and prevalence of stroke is likely to rise with the aging global population.[2] This increase will require all facets of health care to focus on optimizing stroke care and outcomes.[3] Particular emphasis will be on the recovery of function (performance), prevention of secondary complications, reduction of caregiver burden, and the improvement of overall quality of life.

Physical medicine and rehabilitation, or physiatry, is the medical specialty that strives to facilitate recovery, enhance or restore functional ability, anticipate long-term complications, and improve the quality of life for those with physical impairments or disabilities.[4,5] The scope of practice is so broad that it is often said that physiatry

a Department of Rehabilitation Medicine, Weill Cornell Medical College, 525 East 68th Street, Baker 16, New York, NY 10065, USA; b Department of Rehabilitation Medicine, Columbia University College of Physicians and Surgeons, New York Presbyterian Hospital, 180 Fort Washington Avenue, HP1-199, New York, NY 10032, USA
* Corresponding author.
E-mail address: Lel9053@med.cornell.edu

Med Clin N Am 104 (2020) 199–211
https://doi.org/10.1016/j.mcna.2019.11.002
0025-7125/20/© 2019 Elsevier Inc. All rights reserved.

medical.theclinics.com

intersects with virtually every other branch of medicine. In addition, physiatry consultants can aide in managing symptoms and directing early rehabilitation efforts after neurologic and orthopedic injury.[6–10] Stroke rehabilitation can be divided into the acute, postacute, and chronic phases. In each phase, the needs of the patient and the focus of rehabilitation team are different. Some of the differences and opportunities for collaborative care are highlighted in this article. Many of the issues in the chronic phase are addressed in the section on management of common impairments.

Understanding Neurorehabilitation

It was once thought that there was no regenerative ability in the brain or spinal cord and no new cells could be generated nor new connections formulated; thereby limiting potential for functional recovery after injury.[11] This dogma has fallen out of favor and replaced by a model of neuroplasticity resulting from active exercise.[12] Within the sphere of rehabilitation, this has resulted in widespread use of the complementary strategies of compensatory and restorative (remedial, therapeutic) approaches to stroke recovery.[12]

A compensatory approach adapts behavior, the individual, or the environment to find a new way to perform and complete a task. Examples include the using of a cane in the setting of hemiparesis resulting in safer walking, installing a ramp in lieu of stairs, or learning to use the left arm to complete tasks in the setting of right hemiparesis.

Conversely, restorative therapies attempt to develop new or repair damaged neural networks through active exercise with the goal of recovering function and independence. Structured task-specific and intensive exercises in a controlled therapy environment aims to minimize deficits in mobility and ADLs.[12] An example of this type of rehabilitation is constraint-induced movement therapy during which the unaffected limb is restrained and the patient is forced to use the hemiparetic limb during task-oriented exercises.[13,14]

Typically, both approaches, compensatory and restorative, are used simultaneously, as the timeframe for the latter is weeks to months. The rehabilitation team chooses the appropriate therapies to enhance performance and facilitate recovery.[15,16]

Acute Phase of Stroke Rehabilitation

Data strongly suggest a benefit to starting stroke rehabilitation as soon as the patient is medically stable and capable.[17] Within hours, the multidisciplinary rehabilitation team will initiate a detailed assessment to determine the extent of functional impairment and provide education for the patient and caregivers about appropriate next steps in the rehabilitation process.[17,18] However, therapeutic interventions at this early stage may be limited by active medical issues, activity restrictions, or mental status.[19,20]

Early mobilization is defined as trained rehabilitation therapists and nursing staff assisting the patient with task-specific activities, such as active sitting, standing, and walking. It was found that early and regular mobilization in short sessions within 24 hours of diagnosis of stroke predicted better outcomes at 3 months. However, longer duration therapy sessions led to an increase in adverse events.[21] In this acute setting, physiatry is beneficial in guiding the rehabilitation processes and providing education on the goals of mobilization, the next phase of recovery, and barriers to discharge.[22]

Rehabilitation physicians and therapists also may uncover symptoms that are not readily apparent but that are functionally significant and prognostic, such as neglect and hemianopsia. Given that prognosis can impact the intensity and duration of rehabilitation services provided, it is important to monitor for positive and negative factors.[23] Poor prognostic factors include coma at onset of stroke, urinary incontinence, poor cognitive function, severe hemiplegia, perceptual and spatial disorders, and depression.[24,25] Conversely, an independent level of function before stroke is a positive factor, and full assessment of premorbid function is recommended.[26]

The use of neuropharmacologic strategies in combination with exercise may potentially accelerate or augment the recovery process. Dopamine and catecholamine agonists, and anticholinergic antagonist have shown limited degrees of efficacy to treat aphasia after stroke.[27] Similarly, results of these agents for motor recovery after stroke have been mixed.[28] The selective serotonin reuptake inhibitor (SSRI) fluoxetine after the FLAME trial revealed improved upper and lower extremity motor recovery and decreased rates of depression after ischemic stroke.[29] However, more recent data, using different outcome measures, has cast some doubt on the effect of SSRIs on recovery, and further studies are under way. Nevertheless, the desire to reduce neural inflammation, modify synaptic function, and restore cortical network balance continues to fuel pharmacologic study.[30]

There are also classes of medications that can impede stroke recovery. These include first-generation neuroleptic medications (and metoclopramide), benzodiazepines, central adrenergic agonists, and the antiseizure agents phenytoin and phenobarbital. These medications should be considered relatively contraindicated for, at least, the first several months after stroke.[31] In addition, these medications are often cognitively sedating.[28]

Postacute Phase

Postacute rehabilitation services are designed to facilitate recovery, minimize complications, and maximize function following stroke. The most common settings are an inpatient rehabilitation facility, skilled nursing facility, long-term acute care hospital, home-based services, and outpatient services. These settings are best characterized by the intensity of rehabilitation services and degree of medical oversight provided.[3] Some patients will qualify for home health care agency (HHCAs) to provide skilled nursing care and rehabilitation therapy, as well as limited assistance with daily tasks provided by home health aides. These services may also be performed in assisted living facilities or other group home settings.[3]

REHABILITATION OF COMMON POSTSTROKE IMPAIRMENTS
Bowel and Bladder Dysfunction

Neurogenic bladder and bowel dysfunction are defined as any alteration in the controlled, predictable, and socially acceptable elimination of bodily waste after neurologic injury. Common manifestation includes impaired bladder, bowel, and sphincter control.[32–35] In other instances, there is an inability to physically get to a bathroom to void. A full assessment includes a detailed event history, routine laboratory tests, and potential urology and/or gastroenterology referral when more detailed evaluation is needed.[33] Medication management can be effective in treating some causes of urinary dysfunction, but in the setting of stroke certain medications are preferred (**Table 1**). Last, botulinum toxin injection and surgical procedures may need to be considered for symptom management after failure of conservative measures. In this setting, referral to a urologist with experience treating neurologic conditions is warranted.[36–38]

Table 1
Common bladder dysfunction after stroke and treatment options

Type of Incontinence	Common Causes	Common Symptoms	Treatment Options
Detrusor over activity (idiopathic or neurogenic)	Urinary tract infection, stroke, other neurologic disorders	Urinary urgency, frequency	Anticholinergics: oxybutynin, tolterodine, trospium
			Intravesical botulinum toxin injection, sacral nerve stimulation
Overflow incontinence	Neurogenic bladder, fecal impaction, benign prostatic hyperplasia	Poor stream, incomplete emptying	Alpha-adrenergic blocker: doxazosin, prazosin 5-alpha-reductase inhibitors: finasteride

Cognitive Impairments

Stroke is commonly associated with physical impairments and is less recognized as the second leading cause of impaired cognition and dementia.[39] Approximately 30% of stroke survivors develop dementia within 1 year of the onset of their stroke.[40,41] Even minor strokes may affect cognition and executive functions, and there is emerging evidence to suggest that transient ischemic attacks also may be associated with impaired cognition.[42]

The areas most affected are memory, language and communication, orientation, attention, and executive function. These impairments impact the patient's ability to perform ADLs, and in the case of younger stroke survivors, will often affect their chance of returning to work (RTW).[43–45] In addition, although physical impairments are expected to improve, there is often a worsening in the progression of poststroke cognitive deficits.

Cognitive rehabilitation therapy (CRT) is a broad term used to describe treatments done in a variety of settings to address cognitive impairments. It typically begins with an evaluation by physiatry and neuropsychology, and is followed by treatment by speech language pathologist (SLP) and occupational therapy (OT) to address the communication and functional ramifications, respectively. The major goal of CRT is to help patients with cognitive impairments function fully either by focusing on improving the impairments (such as retraining memory function), and/or establish new patterns of cognitive activity. A secondary goal is to provide compensation strategies to cope with the disabling impact of the impairment.

Language and Communication Impairments

Aphasia

Aphasia is a disorder of language resulting from damage to the language-dominant hemisphere of the brain (usually the left side) that impairs comprehension and/or expression of both oral and written language. It is generally classified by fluency of verbal output, auditory comprehension, naming, and repetition. Nonfluent aphasia is characterized by slow and labored verbal output of short phases (no more than a few words) with difficulty in initiating speech. Fluent aphasia is characterized by a more normal speech pattern with adequate phrase length and easy articulation, but lacks content or meaning. These deficits may further disrupt social interaction and interpersonal relationships.[46] Patients with nonfluent aphasia tend to have a poorer prognosis than those with fluent aphasia. Recovery was initially believed to occur within 3 to 6 months after stroke, but new literature suggests that patients may continue to benefit from rehabilitation even in the chronic stages.[47,48]

Treatment by SLP may be done one-on-one or in a group setting with the main goals of therapy is to improve speech, comprehension, communication, and the ability to read and write.

Motor speech disorders

Motor speech disorders (MSDs) include apraxia of speech and dysarthria. Apraxia is an inability to plan or program sensorimotor commands necessary for directing movements required for normal speech (an impairment in "motor planning"). It may be present with or without dysarthria or aphasia.[49–51]

Dysarthria affects 20% to 30% of stroke survivors. It is an articulation deficit characterized by slow, weak, imprecise, and/or uncoordinated movements of the oral musculature resulting from disturbance in neuromuscular control. This manifests as reduced intelligibility of speech. Unlike aphasia, there are no impairments with thoughts, memory, or word finding.[49]

As in the case of language disorders, MSDs are also treated by an SLP. Treatment focuses on strategies and exercises to maximize the clarity of speech and cope with social interaction.

Neglect Syndrome

Visuo-spatial neglect is a disorder of visual and spatial attention in which the patient does not respond to or acknowledge sensory stimuli presented to the body contralateral to the brain lesion. In extreme cases, patients may also fail to acknowledge their own body parts on the affected side. Neglect has been reported in 43% of patients with right hemispheric damage and 17% of those with impairments on the left, and can negatively impact the patient's quality of life, mobility, and safety awareness, and increase falls risk.[52,53] Encouragingly, neglect following stroke usually improves within a few weeks after onset, although a subset of patients will require ongoing therapeutic interventions from OT and physical therapy (PT).[54–58]

Poststroke Dysphagia

Poststroke dysphagia represents a disturbance in the flow of food from the mouth to esophagus, and is said to affect anywhere from 25% to 65% of patients depending on the assessment method used.[59–61] The impairment results from abnormal functioning of the muscles of the mouth, pharynx, and upper esophageal sphincter. It may clinically manifest as food and/or drink exiting the patient's nose, or oxygen desaturation, persistent cough, and/or a change in voice quality during meals. "Pocketing," or accumulation of food on the weak side of the mouth may also be observed. Dysphagia may have a less obvious presentation in which the only complaint is the sensation of food being stuck in the throat. Even more concerning, silent aspiration may also occur, in which there is no cough, complaint, or overt display of aspiration.[59,62,63]

The medical complications associated with dysphagia include aspiration pneumonia, malnutrition, dehydration, prolonged hospitalization, and mortality.[64] Dysphagia also can reduce the joy associated with eating and result in increased anxiety and panic episodes surrounding mealtimes.[65–67]

Effective treatment begins with a thorough history to help determine the type of dysphagia. Video fluoroscopic swallow study, also known as the modified barium swallow (MBS) study, is often considered the assessment of choice. SLP provides the patient with various consistencies of food and liquid mixed with barium, which is visualized on radiographs for evidence of swallowing dysfunction. Another evaluation is the fiberoptic endoscopic evaluation of swallowing test, in which the SLP passes an endoscope trans-nasally for direct visualization of swallowing.

Effective treatment of poststroke dysphagia requires an interdisciplinary team approach with SLP, OT, nursing, and physiatry, as well as involvement of the patient and family. Treatment strategies used include strengthening exercises, compensatory strategies during swallowing, and changes in food type, amount, and consistency. In some cases, supervision during meals may be required.[68]

Musculoskeletal Disorders and Pain Syndromes

Stroke survivors may experience pain resulting from central and peripheral mechanisms, as well as psychological factors. Symptoms may occur immediately after stroke and for some may continue indefinitely.[69] Common etiologies include poststroke pain syndromes, hemiplegic shoulder pain, shoulder subluxation, rotator cuff injury, arthralgia, osteoarthritis, impingement syndrome, bicipital tendonitis, complex regional pain syndrome, heterotopic ossification, spasticity, and joint contractures.[70] It is important to realize that patients may also experience symptoms from premorbid musculoskeletal issues as seen in the general population.[71] Physiatrist are uniquely trained to provide comprehensive management of pain, neurologic, and musculoskeletal complications seen in stroke survivors.

Central poststroke pain

Central poststroke pain (CPSP) is a chronic neuropathic disorder typically experienced within the first month after stroke but ranging from 1 week to 10 years. Prevalence varies from 7% to 35% and the mechanism is not well understood. Pain may be intermittent or constant, with sensory abnormalities, and is described as burning, aching, icy, pricking, and lacerating.[72]

As is typical of neuropathic pain, patients with CPSP respond poorly to conventional analgesia and are often treated with various types of psychoactive and neuromodulating agents. Commonly used pharmacologic agents include tricyclic antidepressants, SSRIs, serotonin norepinephrine reuptake inhibitors, membrane stabilizing agents such as gabapentin and pregabalin, anticonvulsants, corticosteroids, and opioids. Because of the challenging nature of this pain, medications are often used in combination.[73] One nonpharmacologic approach is the prescription of exercise therapy to improve strength, flexibility, and function.[69,74,75]

Poststroke shoulder pain

Poststroke shoulder pain is a term used broadly to describe shoulder pain on the weak limb in a person with hemiplegic stroke. It is present in 25% of stroke survivors.[71,76–79] Etiologies may include rotator cuff injury, subluxation, shoulder-hand syndrome, myofascial pain syndrome, adhesive capsulitis, spasticity, and contracture.[69] Pain can develop as early as 2 weeks after stroke but is more commonly seen at 2 to 3 months.[76] Treatment involves effective pain control with similar agents used to treat CPSP, subacromial steroid injection, physical modalities, and a program of rehabilitation.

Mood Disorders Following Stroke

Neuropsychiatric disorders associated with stroke include depression, anxiety disorder, pseudobulbar affect, anosognosia, and many others. Of these, depression is the most frequent to occur following stroke and has been shown to negatively impact the stroke survivor's functional outcome, response to rehabilitation, and quality of life.[80–83] The incidence of post stroke depression (PSD) has been reported at 30% and the risk increases in patients with a prior history of anxiety or depression.[84,85] Treatment includes early psychiatry evaluation and the use of antidepressants. Cognitive behavioral therapy has been shown to be the most effective psychotherapeutic intervention.

Poststoke Fatigue

Poststoke fatigue is a poorly understood, multidimensional, emotional, and cognitive experience in which patients often describe a feeling of exhaustion and a lack of energy and effort. Fatigue is one of the more prevalent symptoms after stroke, with frequency ranging from 29% to 77%, and its presence may inhibit participation and progress in rehabilitation.[86–89] The symptom often develops after physical or mental activity and usually improves with rest.[87,90]

Treatment approaches include the use of antidepressants (SSRIs), modafinil, and counseling to help ameliorate the depressive symptoms associated with fatigue.[91–93] Because impaired sleep may coexist with poststroke fatigue, patients may benefit from education in good sleep hygiene and the benefits of regular exercise.[94,95] When interventions are ineffective, patients should manage their activities and plan for rest breaks.[96,97]

Spasticity and Joint Contracture

Spasticity is disoriented sensory-motor control, resulting from an upper motor neuron lesion, presenting as intermittent or sustained involuntary activation of muscles.[98–100] The presentation of spasticity after stroke is variable, and approximately 30% of patients with stroke develop spasticity in the paretic limb. Spasticity is commonly found in the shoulder, flexor muscles of the upper arm (elbow, wrist, and fingers), and extensor muscles of the lower limb (knee and ankle). If untreated, spasticity may lead to pain, contracture, worsened mobility, poor quality of life, and increased caregiver burden.[101] Early detection and management of spasticity may help mitigate these complications.

Treatment often includes range of motion with PT or OT, stretching, modalities, and oral antispasm agents, such as baclofen, tizanidine, and dantrolene. Physiatric management includes the administration of botulinum toxin injections, neurolysis with phenol or alcohol, and the use of intrathecal baclofen.[102] In addition, in the presence of true joint contracture that limits function, pain-free movement, and hygiene, a surgical consultation may be warranted.

Sexual Dysfunction

After a stroke, approximately 57% to 75% of patients suffer from some form of sexual dysfunction.[103,104] Common complaints include decline in libido, decrease in coital frequency, reduction in vaginal lubrication and orgasm in women, and poor or failed erection and ejaculation in men.[104,105]

Pharmacologic management is similar to that for patients with sexual dysfunction in the general population. Counseling by the multidisciplinary team aims to assess existing sexual issues, provides education, and offers support to ensure a safe return to sexual activity after a stroke.[106–108]

Employment and Return to Work

Although the incidence of stroke in significantly lower in young adults, this population stands to lose more economically because they are disabled in their most productive, working years.[109,110] To help determine if the stroke survivor is able to safely RTW, a referral may be made to OT or PT for a functional capacity evaluation.[111]

Driving After Stroke

Due to the motor, visual, and cognitive impairments that accompany strokes, some survivors may have limitations in their driving ability. Health providers should refer to their state regulations for guidance about requirements for return to driving. Patients can be referred to specialized centers where PT or OT assist with screening and driver evaluation. Neuropsychology evaluation can aid in determining an individual's capacity to drive safely after stroke.[112,113]

SUMMARY

This article summarizes the scope and breadth of stroke rehabilitation. There is much work to be done to improve access to the available rehabilitation services, improve coordination of care across health care systems, and to secure the most desirable poststroke outcomes. Prevention, early recognition, and early intervention will likely limit the severity and cost of these poststroke conditions.[114] An understanding of the significance of poststroke complications on the part of internists and family practice physicians will likely drive more streamlined care, quality, and outcome-based interventions, better integration of technologies, and the re-imagination of services provided.

DISCLOSURE

The authors have nothing to disclose.

REFERENCES

1. Benjamin EJ, Virani SS, Callaway CW, et al. Heart disease and stroke statistics-2018 update: a report from the American Heart Association. Circulation 2018; 137(12):e67–492.
2. Hall MJ, Levant S, DeFrances CJ. Hospitalization for stroke in U.S. hospitals, 1989-2009. NCHS Data Brief 2012;(95):1–8.
3. Winstein CJ, Stein J, Arena R, et al. Guidelines for adult stroke rehabilitation and recovery: a guideline for healthcare professionals from the American Heart Association/American Stroke Association. Stroke 2016;47(6):e98–169.
4. Frederickson M, Cannon NL. The role of the rehabilitation physician in the postacute continuum. Arch Phys Med Rehabil 1995;76(12 Suppl):Sc5–9.
5. Bartels MN. Physiatry as a leader for postacute care in integrated healthcare systems. Am J Phys Med Rehabil 2019;98(4):311–8.
6. Greiss C, Yonclas PP, Jasey N, et al. Presence of a dedicated trauma center physiatrist improves functional outcomes following traumatic brain injury. J Trauma Acute Care Surg 2016;80(1):70–5.
7. Sepulveda F, Baerga L, Micheo W. The role of physiatry in regenerative medicine: the past, the present, and future challenges. PM R 2015;7(4 Suppl):S76–80.
8. O'Dell MW, Dunning K, Kluding P, et al. Response and prediction of improvement in gait speed from functional electrical stimulation in persons with poststroke drop foot. PM R 2014;6(7):587–601 [quiz: 601].
9. Subramanian SK. Virtual reality in rehabilitation—using technology to enhance function. PM R 2018;10(11):1221–2.
10. Belagaje SR. Stroke rehabilitation. Continuum (Minneap Minn) 2017;23(1, Cerebrovascular Disease):238–53.
11. Stahnisch FW, Nitsch R. Santiago Ramon y Cajal's concept of neuronal plasticity: the ambiguity lives on. Trends Neurosci 2002;25(11):589–91.

12. Mark VW, Taub E, Morris DM. Neuroplasticity and constraint-induced movement therapy. Eura Medicophys 2006;42(3):269–84.
13. Uswatte G, Taub E, Morris D, et al. Contribution of the shaping and restraint components of constraint-induced movement therapy to treatment outcome. NeuroRehabilitation 2006;21(2):147–56.
14. Brogardh C, Sjolund BH. Constraint-induced movement therapy in patients with stroke: a pilot study on effects of small group training and of extended mitt use. Clin Rehabil 2006;20(3):218–27.
15. Partridge C, Edwards S. The bases of practice—neurological physiotherapy. Physiother Res Int 1996;1(3):205–8.
16. Langhorne P, Coupar F, Pollock A. Motor recovery after stroke: a systematic review. Lancet Neurol 2009;8(8):741–54.
17. Miller EL, Murray L, Richards L, et al. Comprehensive overview of nursing and interdisciplinary rehabilitation care of the stroke patient: a scientific statement from the American Heart Association. Stroke 2010;41(10):2402–48.
18. Prvu Bettger J, Alexander KP, Dolor RJ, et al. Transitional care after hospitalization for acute stroke or myocardial infarction: a systematic review. Ann Intern Med 2012;157(6):407–16.
19. Witcher R, Stoerger L, Dzierba AL, et al. Effect of early mobilization on sedation practices in the neurosciences intensive care unit: a preimplementation and postimplementation evaluation. J Crit Care 2015;30(2):344–7.
20. Needham DM, Korupolu R. Rehabilitation quality improvement in an intensive care unit setting: implementation of a quality improvement model. Top Stroke Rehabil 2010;17(4):271–81.
21. Bernhardt J, Dewey H, Thrift A, et al. A very early rehabilitation trial for stroke (AVERT): phase II safety and feasibility. Stroke 2008;39(2):390–6.
22. Momosaki R, Kakuda W, Yamada N, et al. Impact of board-certificated physiatrists on rehabilitation outcomes in elderly patients after hip fracture: an observational study using the Japan Rehabilitation Database. Geriatr Gerontol Int 2016;16(8):963–8.
23. Jongbloed L. Prediction of function after stroke: a critical review. Stroke 1986; 17(4):765–76.
24. DeJong G, Branch LG. Predicting the stroke patient's ability to live independently. Stroke 1982;13(5):648–55.
25. Chen P, Hreha K, Kong Y, et al. Impact of spatial neglect on stroke rehabilitation: evidence from the setting of an inpatient rehabilitation facility. Arch Phys Med Rehabil 2015;96(8):1458–66.
26. Hay CC, Graham J, Pappadis MR, et al. The impact of one's sex and social living situation on rehabilitation outcomes following a stroke. Am J Phys Med Rehabil 2020;99(1):48–55.
27. Ashtary F, Janghorbani M, Chitsaz A, et al. A randomized, double-blind trial of bromocriptine efficacy in nonfluent aphasia after stroke. Neurology 2006; 66(6):914–6.
28. Keser Z, Francisco GE. Neuropharmacology of poststroke motor and speech recovery. Phys Med Rehabil Clin N Am 2015;26(4):671–89.
29. Chollet F, Tardy J, Albucher JF, et al. Fluoxetine for motor recovery after acute ischaemic stroke (FLAME): a randomised placebo-controlled trial. Lancet Neurol 2011;10(2):123–30.
30. Lin DJ, Finklestein SP, Cramer SC. New directions in treatments targeting stroke recovery. Stroke 2018;49(12):3107–14.

31. Goldstein LB, Bullman S. Differential effects of haloperidol and clozapine on motor recovery after sensorimotor cortex injury in rats. Neurorehabil Neural Repair 2002;16(4):321–5.

32. Karsenty G, Reitz A, Wefer B, et al. Understanding detrusor sphincter dyssynergia–significance of chronology. Urology 2005;66(4):763–8.

33. Stohrer M, Goepel M, Kondo A, et al. The standardization of terminology in neurogenic lower urinary tract dysfunction: with suggestions for diagnostic procedures. International Continence Society Standardization Committee. Neurourol Urodyn 1999;18(2):139–58.

34. John G, Primmaz S, Crichton S, et al. Urinary incontinence and indwelling urinary catheters as predictors of death after new-onset stroke: a report of the South London Stroke Register. J Stroke Cerebrovasc Dis 2018;27(1):118–24.

35. Thomas LH, Coupe J, Cross LD, et al. Interventions for treating urinary incontinence after stroke in adults. Stroke 2019;50(8):e226–7.

36. Thomas LH, Coupe J, Cross LD, et al. Interventions for treating urinary incontinence after stroke in adults. Cochrane Database Syst Rev 2019;(2):CD004462.

37. Lorish TR, Sandin KJ, Roth EJ, et al. Stroke rehabilitation. 3. Rehabilitation evaluation and management. Arch Phys Med Rehabil 1994;75(5 Spec No):S47–51.

38. Engler TM, Dourado CC, Amancio TG, et al. Stroke: bowel dysfunction in patients admitted for rehabilitation. Open Nurs J 2014;8:43–7.

39. Al-Qazzaz NK, Ali SH, Ahmad SA, et al. Cognitive impairment and memory dysfunction after a stroke diagnosis: a post-stroke memory assessment. Neuropsychiatr Dis Treat 2014;10:1677–91.

40. Cullen B, O'Neill B, Evans JJ, et al. A review of screening tests for cognitive impairment. J Neurol Neurosurg Psychiatry 2007;78(8):790–9.

41. Mijajlovic MD, Pavlovic A, Brainin M, et al. Post-stroke dementia—a comprehensive review. BMC Med 2017;15(1):11.

42. van Rooij FG, Kessels RP, Richard E, et al. Cognitive impairment in transient ischemic attack patients: a systematic review. Cerebrovasc Dis 2016; 42(1–2):1–9.

43. Fride Y, Adamit T, Maeir A, et al. What are the correlates of cognition and participation to return to work after first ever mild stroke? Top Stroke Rehabil 2015; 22(5):317–25.

44. QUERI Polytrauma/Blast-Related Injuries [Internet], Fiscal year 2010 VA utilization report for Iraq and Afghanistan war veterans diagnosed with TBI. Minneapolis (MN): Minneapolis VA Health Care System; 2012. Available at. http://www. queri.research.va.gov/ptbri/docs/FY10-TBI-Diagnosis-HCU-Report.pdf.

45. das Nair R, Cogger H, Worthington E, et al. Cognitive rehabilitation for memory deficits after stroke. Cochrane Database Syst Rev 2016;(9):CD002293.

46. Patel S, Oishi K, Wright A, et al. Right hemisphere regions critical for expression of emotion through prosody. Front Neurol 2018;9:224.

47. Doogan C, Dignam J, Copland D, et al. Aphasia recovery: when, how and who to treat? Curr Neurol Neurosci Rep 2018;18(12):90.

48. Fama ME, Turkeltaub PE. Treatment of poststroke aphasia: current practice and new directions. Semin Neurol 2014;34(5):504–13.

49. Duffy J. Motor speech disorders: substrates, differential diagnosis, and management. 3rd edition. St Louis (MO): Elsevier; 2013.

50. Mitchell C, Bowen A, Tyson S, et al. Interventions for dysarthria due to stroke and other adult-acquired, non-progressive brain injury. Cochrane Database Syst Rev 2017;(1):CD002088.

51. Kwon YG, Do KH, Park SJ, et al. Effect of repetitive transcranial magnetic stimulation on patients with dysarthria after subacute stroke. Ann Rehabil Med 2015; 39(5):793–9.

52. Halligan PW, Robertson I. Spatial neglect: a clinical handbook for diagnosis and treatment. New York: Psychology Press; 1999.

53. Buxbaum LJ, Ferraro MK, Veramonti T, et al. Hemispatial neglect: subtypes, neuroanatomy, and disability. Neurology 2004;62(5):749–56.

54. Parton A, Malhotra P, Husain M. Hemineglect. J Neurol Neurosurg Psychiatry 2004;75:13–21.

55. Kwon JS. Therapeutic intervention for visuo-spatial neglect after stroke: a meta-analysis of randomized controlled trials. Osong Public Health Res Perspect 2018;9(2):59–65.

56. Tsang MH, Sze KH, Fong KN. Occupational therapy treatment with right half-field eye-patching for patients with subacute stroke and unilateral neglect: a randomised controlled trial. Disabil Rehabil 2009;31(8):630–7.

57. Smania N, Fonte C, Picelli A, et al. Effect of eye patching in rehabilitation of hemispatial neglect. Front Hum Neurosci 2013;7:527.

58. Serino A, Barbiani M, Rinaldesi ML, et al. Effectiveness of prism adaptation in neglect rehabilitation: a controlled trial study. Stroke 2009;40(4):1392–8.

59. Ramsey DJ, Smithard DG, Kalra L. Early assessments of dysphagia and aspiration risk in acute stroke patients. Stroke 2003;34(5):1252–7.

60. Gordon C, Hewer RL, Wade DT. Dysphagia in acute stroke. Br Med J (Clin Res Ed) 1987;295(6595):411–4.

61. Smithard DG, O'Neill PA, England RE, et al. The natural history of dysphagia following a stroke. Dysphagia 1997;12(4):188–93.

62. Kidd D, Lawson J, Nesbitt R, et al. Aspiration in acute stroke: a clinical study with videofluoroscopy. Q J Med 1993;86(12):825–9.

63. Daniels SK, Brailey K, Priestly DH, et al. Aspiration in patients with acute stroke. Arch Phys Med Rehabil 1998;79(1):14–9.

64. Cohen DL, Roffe C, Beavan J, et al. Post-stroke dysphagia: a review and design considerations for future trials. Int J Stroke 2016;11(4):399–411.

65. Orlandoni P, Peladic NJ. Health-related quality of life and functional health status questionnaires in oropharyngeal dysphagia. J Aging Res Clin Pract 2016; 5:31–7.

66. Aviv JE, Kim T, Sacco RL, et al. FEESST: a new bedside endoscopic test of the motor and sensory components of swallowing. Ann Otol Rhinol Laryngol 1998; 107(5 Pt 1):378–87.

67. Giammarino C, Adams E, Moriarty C, et al. Safety concerns and multidisciplinary management of the dysphagic patient. Phys Med Rehabil Clin N Am 2012;23(2):335–42.

68. Hinds NP, Wiles CM. Assessment of swallowing and referral to speech and language therapists in acute stroke. QJM 1998;91(12):829–35.

69. Treister AK, Hatch MN, Cramer SC, et al. Demystifying poststroke pain: from etiology to treatment. PM R 2017;9(1):63–75.

70. O'Donnell MJ, Diener HC, Sacco RL, et al. Chronic pain syndromes after ischemic stroke: PRoFESS trial. Stroke 2013;44(5):1238–43.

71. Kendall R. Musculoskeletal problems in stroke survivors. Top Stroke Rehabil 2010;17(3):173–8.

72. Oh H, Seo W. A comprehensive review of central post-stroke pain. Pain Manag Nurs 2015;16(5):804–18.

73. Pickering AE, Thornton SR, Love-Jones SJ, et al. Analgesia in conjunction with normalisation of thermal sensation following deep brain stimulation for central post-stroke pain. Pain 2009;147(1–3):299–304.

74. Mulla SM, Wang L, Khokhar R, et al. Management of central poststroke pain: systematic review of randomized controlled trials. Stroke 2015;46(10):2853–60.

75. Rossi S, Hallett M, Rossini PM, et al. Safety, ethical considerations, and application guidelines for the use of transcranial magnetic stimulation in clinical practice and research. Clin Neurophysiol 2009;120(12):2008–39.

76. Paolucci S, Martinuzzi A, Scivoletto G, et al. Assessing and treating pain associated with stroke, multiple sclerosis, cerebral palsy, spinal cord injury and spasticity. Evidence and recommendations from the Italian Consensus Conference on Pain in Neurorehabilitation. Eur J Phys Rehabil Med 2016;52(6):827–40.

77. Liporaci FM, Mourani MM, Riberto M. The myofascial component of the pain in the painful shoulder of the hemiplegic patient. Clinics (Sao Paulo) 2019;74:e905.

78. Garrison DW, Foreman RD. Decreased activity of spontaneous and noxiously evoked dorsal horn cells during transcutaneous electrical nerve stimulation (TENS). Pain 1994;58(3):309–15.

79. Rah UW, Yoon SH, Moon DJ, et al. Subacromial corticosteroid injection on post-stroke hemiplegic shoulder pain: a randomized, triple-blind, placebo-controlled trial. Arch Phys Med Rehabil 2012;93(6):949–56.

80. Robinson RG, Jorge RE. Post-stroke depression: a review. Am J Psychiatry 2016;173(3):221–31.

81. House A, Dennis M, Mogridge L, et al. Mood disorders in the year after first stroke. Br J Psychiatry 1991;158:83–92.

82. Santos M, Kovari E, Gold G, et al. The neuroanatomical model of post-stroke depression: towards a change of focus? J Neurol Sci 2009;283(1–2):158–62.

83. Rajashekaran P, Pai K, Thunga R, et al. Post-stroke depression and lesion location: a hospital based cross-sectional study. Indian J Psychiatry 2013;55(4):343–8.

84. De Ryck A, Brouns R, Geurden M, et al. Risk factors for poststroke depression: identification of inconsistencies based on a systematic review. J Geriatr Psychiatry Neurol 2014;27(3):147–58.

85. Starkstein SE, Hayhow BD. Treatment of post-stroke depression. Curr Treat Options Neurol 2019;21(7):31.

86. Glader EL, Stegmayr B, Asplund K. Poststroke fatigue: a 2-year follow-up study of stroke patients in Sweden. Stroke 2002;33(5):1327–33.

87. Acciarresi M, Bogousslavsky J, Paciaroni M. Post-stroke fatigue: epidemiology, clinical characteristics and treatment. Eur Neurol 2014;72(5–6):255–61.

88. van der Werf SP, van den Broek HL, Anten HW, et al. Experience of severe fatigue long after stroke and its relation to depressive symptoms and disease characteristics. Eur Neurol 2001;45(1):28–33.

89. Schepers VP, Visser-Meily AM, Ketelaar M, et al. Poststroke fatigue: course and its relation to personal and stroke-related factors. Arch Phys Med Rehabil 2006; 87(2):184–8.

90. Staub F, Bogousslavsky J. Fatigue after stroke: a major but neglected issue. Cerebrovasc Dis 2001;12(2):75–81.

91. Mead G, Bernhardt J, Kwakkel G. Stroke: physical fitness, exercise, and fatigue. Stroke Res Treat 2012;2012:632531.

92. Puchta AE. Why am I so tired after my stroke? J Vasc Interv Neurol 2008; 1(2):63–4.

93. Bivard A, Lillicrap T, Krishnamurthy V, et al. MIDAS (modafinil in debilitating fatigue after stroke): a randomized, double-blind, placebo-controlled, cross-over trial. Stroke 2017;48(5):1293–8.
94. Davies DP, Rodgers H, Walshaw D, et al. Snoring, daytime sleepiness and stroke: a case-control study of first-ever stroke. J Sleep Res 2003;12(4):313–8.
95. Passier PE, Post MW, van Zandvoort MJ, et al. Predicting fatigue 1 year after aneurysmal subarachnoid hemorrhage. J Neurol 2011;258(6):1091–7.
96. Broomfield NM, Laidlaw K, Hickabottom E, et al. Post-stroke depression: the case for augmented, individually tailored cognitive behavioural therapy. Clin Psychol Psychother 2011;18(3):202–17.
97. Barbour VL, Mead GE. Fatigue after stroke: the patient's perspective. Stroke Res Treat 2012;2012:863031.
98. Bhimani R, Anderson L. Clinical understanding of spasticity: implications for practice. Rehabil Res Pract 2014;2014:279175.
99. Welmer AK, Widen Holmqvist L, Sommerfeld DK. Location and severity of spasticity in the first 1-2 weeks and at 3 and 18 months after stroke. Eur J Neurol 2010;17(5):720–5.
100. Francisco GE, McGuire JR. Poststroke spasticity management. Stroke 2012; 43(11):3132–6.
101. Wissel J, Verrier M, Simpson DM, et al. Post-stroke spasticity: predictors of early development and considerations for therapeutic intervention. PM R 2015;7(1):60–7.
102. Marciniak C. Poststroke hypertonicity: upper limb assessment and treatment. Top Stroke Rehabil 2011;18(3):179–94.
103. Korpelainen JT, Nieminen P, Myllyla VV. Sexual functioning among stroke patients and their spouses. Stroke 1999;30(4):715–9.
104. Monga TN, Lawson JS, Inglis J. Sexual dysfunction in stroke patients. Arch Phys Med Rehabil 1986;67(1):19–22.
105. Boldrini P, Basaglia N, Calanca MC. Sexual changes in hemiparetic patients. Arch Phys Med Rehabil 1991;72(3):202–7.
106. Ng L, Sansom J, Zhang N, et al. Effectiveness of a structured sexual rehabilitation programme following stroke: a randomized controlled trial. J Rehabil Med 2017;49(4):333–40.
107. Lue TF, Giuliano F, Montorsi F, et al. Summary of the recommendations on sexual dysfunctions in men. J Sex Med 2004;1(1):6–23.
108. Byrne M, Doherty S, Fridlund BG, et al. Sexual counselling for sexual problems in patients with cardiovascular disease. Cochrane Database Syst Rev 2016;(2):CD010988.
109. Smajlovic D. Strokes in young adults: epidemiology and prevention. Vasc Health Risk Manag 2015;11:157–64.
110. van der Kemp J, Kruithof WJ, Nijboer TCW, et al. Return to work after mild-to-moderate stroke: work satisfaction and predictive factors. Neuropsychol Rehabil 2019;29(4):638–53.
111. Chen JJ. Functional capacity evaluation & disability. Iowa Orthop J 2007;27: 121–7.
112. Wolfe PL, Lehockey KA. Neuropsychological assessment of driving capacity. Arch Clin Neuropsychol 2016;31(6):517–29.
113. George S, Crotty M, Gelinas I, et al. Rehabilitation for improving automobile driving after stroke. Cochrane Database Syst Rev 2014;(2):CD008357.
114. Tong X, George MG, Gillespie C, et al. Trends in hospitalizations and cost associated with stroke by age, United States 2003-2012. Int J Stroke 2016;11(8): 874–81.

Traumatic Brain Injury
An Overview of Epidemiology, Pathophysiology, and Medical Management

Allison Capizzi, MD[a], Jean Woo, MD[b],
Monica Verduzco-Gutierrez, MD[c],*

KEYWORDS

- Traumatic brain injury • TBI • Head injury • Acquired brain injury • Concussion
- Disorders of consciousness

KEY POINTS

- Traumatic brain injury (TBI) is gaining more attention because of long-term effects as well as increasing rates of brain injury driven by emergency department visits.
- Understanding the severity of TBI helps both with prognosis of functional recovery and in anticipating patients' rehabilitation needs.
- Medical complications are common after moderate and severe TBI and should be considered and addressed by the treating physician.
- There is a high rate of misdiagnosis in patients with severe TBI and disorders of consciousness; therefore, it is imperative to refer these patients to specialized multidisciplinary rehabilitation teams to optimize diagnosis, prognosis, and management.

The goal of this article is to provide a general review of the epidemiology, acute care, and chronic management of adult patients with traumatic brain injuries (TBI). This text was created for providers practicing outside of physical medicine and rehabilitation (PM&R). The medical and rehabilitation management of moderate to severe TBI is the focus of this article, with a brief discussion of the management of mild injuries.

[a] Department of Physical Medicine and Rehabilitation, McGovern Medical School, The University of Texas Health Science Center at Houston, 1333 Moursund Street, Houston, TX 77030, USA; [b] H. Ben Taub Department of Physical Medicine and Rehabilitation, Baylor College of Medicine, 7200 Cambridge St. Houston, TX 77030, USA; [c] Department of Physical Medicine and Rehabilitation, Brain Injury and Stroke Programs, McGovern Medical School, The University of Texas Health Science Center at Houston, TIRR Memorial Hermann Hospital, 1333 Moursund Street, Houston, TX 77030, USA
* Corresponding author.
E-mail address: Monica.verduzco-gutierrez@uth.tmc.edu

Med Clin N Am 104 (2020) 213–238
https://doi.org/10.1016/j.mcna.2019.11.001
0025-7125/20/© 2019 Elsevier Inc. All rights reserved.

medical.theclinics.com

DEFINITIONS

According to the Centers for Disease Control and Prevention (CDC), a TBI is caused by a bump, blow, or jolt to the head, or a penetrating head injury that disrupts the normal function of the brain. Traumatic impact injuries can be defined as closed (nonpenetrating) or open (penetrating).[1,2]

EPIDEMIOLOGY

In 2014, the CDC documented 2.53 million TBI-related emergency department (ED) visits. There were approximately 288,000 TBI-related hospitalizations and 56,800 TBI-related deaths. These data include both adults and children. Older adults aged 75 years and older had the highest rate of TBI-associated ED visits (1682 per 100,000 people) followed by young children 0 to 4 years old (1618.6 per 100,000 people), and last, followed by adolescents and young adults 15 to 24 years old (1010.1 per 100,000 people).[1]

Emergency Department Visits and Deaths

TBI-related ED visits and deaths have increased steadily from 2006 to 2014.[1] This increase may be partially attributed to improved brain injury awareness among providers and more accurate reporting and surveillance methods (**Table 1**).

Table 1 Most common reasons for traumatic brain injury–related hospitalization			
Age Range (years)	**0–17**	**15–44**	**55+**
Mechanism of injury	Falls	MVC	Falls

Modified from Centers for Disease Control and Prevention (2019). Surveillance Report of Traumatic Brain Injury-related Emergency Department Visits, Hospitalizations, and Deaths—United States, 2014. Centers for Disease Control and Prevention, U.S. Department of Health and Human Services.

Deaths

According to 2014 CDC data, the most common causes of TBI-related deaths in descending order are intentional self-harm (32.5%), unintentional falls (28.1%), and motor vehicle crashes (MVC) (18.7%).

Trends in TBI-related deaths tracked from 2006 to 2014 suggest intentional self-harm and unintentional falls are the only monitored categories with increasing incidence (**Table 2**).[1]

Table 2 Most common cause of death by age groups						
Age Range (years)	**0–4**	**15–24**	**25–34**	**45–64**	**65+**	**≥75[a]**
Cause of death	Homicide	MVC	MVC	Intentional self-harm	Falls	MVC

[a] Highest rate of death.

Modified from Centers for Disease Control and Prevention (2019). Surveillance Report of Traumatic Brain Injury-related Emergency Department Visits, Hospitalizations, and Deaths—United States, 2014. Centers for Disease Control and Prevention, U.S. Department of Health and Human Services.

Mechanisms of Injury

The most common mechanisms of injury, in descending order of frequency, include unintentional falls, being unintentionally struck by an object, MVC, assault, other (no mechanism specified), and intentional self-harm.[1]

The Department of Defense identifies TBI as the signature injury of Operation Enduring Freedom and Operation Iraqi Freedom veterans. Blast injuries are a common mechanism of injury associated with this war period.[3]

Severity

Understanding brain injury severity helps with both prognosis of functional recovery and anticipating patients' rehabilitation needs (**Fig. 1**, **Table 3**).

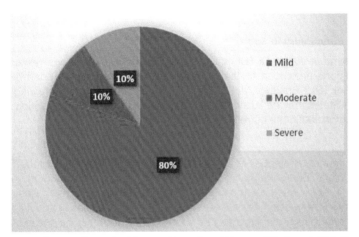

Fig. 1. Severity of TBI in the United States. (*Data from* Wagner AK, Arenth PM, Kwasnica C, et al. Traumatic Brain Injury. In: Cifu DX, editor. Braddom's Physical Medicine and Rehabilitation, 5th edition. Philadelphia: Elsevier; 2016.)

Table 3
Classification of traumatic brain injuries

	GCS[a] (First 24 h)	Loss of Consciousness	Alteration of Consciousness	Imaging	PTA
Mild	13–15	0–30 min	Up to 24 h	Normal	0–1 d
Moderate	9–12	>30 min and <24 h	>24 h	Normal or abnormal	>1 d and <7 d
Severe	3–8	>24 h	>24 h	Normal or abnormal	>7 d

Note: Some institutions use the term "mild complicated TBI" for patients who meet the mild classification by GCS, loss or alteration of consciousness, and posttraumatic amnesia but have abnormal imaging findings, such as a subdural hematoma or depressed skull fracture.[4]

[a] See **Table 4**.

Adapted from Veterans Affairs/Department of Defense. VA/DoD Clinical Practice Guideline for the Management of Concussion-Mild Traumatic Brain Injury. Washington, DC: Veterans Health Administration; 2016, with permission.

Table 4 Glasgow coma scale			
Score	Eye Opening	Verbal	Motor[a]
1	None	None	None
2	To pain	Incomprehensible speech	Extension (decerebrate posturing) to pain
3	To speech	Inappropriate speech	Flexor (decorticate posturing) to pain
4	Spontaneous	Confused	Withdraws to pain
5	–	Oriented	Localizing response
6	–	–	Follows directions

[a] The motor score is the only part of the GCS with prognostic value.
Reprinted with permission from Elsevier (Teasdale G, Jennett B. Assessment of coma and consciousness. A practical scale. Lancet 1974;2(7872):83).

Traumatic Brain Injury in Sports

Current literature suggests TBI makes up 10% to 15% of all sports-related injuries. Collision sports (American football followed by women's soccer) report the highest incidence of TBI.[5] However, adequate reporting systems in other growing sports in the United States may be lacking, potentially leading to overrepresentation or underrepresentation within the current data sets.

Gender

There are gender differences in the epidemiology of TBI. According to the TBI Model System National Database Statistics from 2017, male cases greatly outnumbered female cases, accounting for more than 73% of all TBIs reported.[6] Conversely, in sports-related concussion, female cases outnumber male cases at about a 2:1 ratio.[5] The discrepancy in gender reporting for sports-concussion may be due to cultural differences (women being more willing to report injury than men) or physiologic differences, such as the difference in head-to-neck ratio between men and women.[5] Among older individuals (>65 years), the frequency of TBI is about the same for men and women.[7]

Long-Term Implications

TBI is a leading cause of long-term disability among children and young adults in the United States.[7] Current literature suggests more than 1.1% of the US population is living with a TBI. Of that population, more than 40% of patients with moderate to severe injuries will have long-term disability.[8] Cost estimates are varied, ranging from $56 to $221 billion annually.[2,4,5,7,8] The variation reflects difficulty measuring hidden costs associated with long-term disability, such as lost wages and caregiver expenses.[2,5]

PATHOPHYSIOLOGY

Traumatic injuries disrupt normal cellular function within the brain through direct, rotational, and shear forces. These forces may be present in all severities of injury. Rotational forces disrupt axons within the white matter tracts of the brain, which can lead to diffuse axonal injury. A special MRI technique known as diffusion tensor imaging can evaluate white matter tract damage.[4] In addition, axonal injury results in local swelling, which slows signal transmission. Traumatic injury is also associated with changes in cerebral blood flow, resulting in an initial decrease in blood flow followed by unresponsive vasodilation thought secondary to nitric oxide release in the tissue. This vascular phenomenon is best documented in cases of mild traumatic brain injury (mTBI) in rodent studies.[5,7,9]

The diagram in **Box 1** is a simplified flowchart of the pathophysiology at the cellular level after TBI.

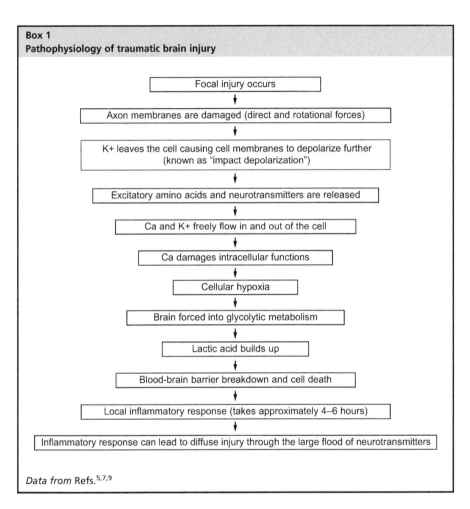

Box 1
Pathophysiology of traumatic brain injury

Focal injury occurs
↓
Axon membranes are damaged (direct and rotational forces)
↓
K+ leaves the cell causing cell membranes to depolarize further (known as "impact depolarization")
↓
Excitatory amino acids and neurotransmitters are released
↓
Ca and K+ freely flow in and out of the cell
↓
Ca damages intracellular functions
↓
Cellular hypoxia
↓
Brain forced into glycolytic metabolism
↓
Lactic acid builds up
↓
Blood-brain barrier breakdown and cell death
↓
Local inflammatory response (takes approximately 4–6 hours)
↓
Inflammatory response can lead to diffuse injury through the large flood of neurotransmitters

Data from Refs.[5,7,9]

Both focal and diffuse injury can occur within the same patient. Focal injury can result from direct or indirect impact. Indirect impact is considered secondary to acceleration-deceleration force. As the brain is surrounded by a layer of cerebral spinal fluid (CSF), force from the direct impact will translate the brain to the opposite side of the skull, resulting in a second impact. Focal injuries are most associated with frontal and temporal lobe damage. Damage to these areas is linked to problems with executive function, impulsivity, and disinhibition (**Table 5**).[5]

Table 5
Primary versus secondary injury

Primary Injury	Secondary Injury
• Direct hit can produce indirect damage through acceleration-deceleration (coup contrecoup) mechanism • Penetrating (open) vs nonpenetrating (closed) • Considered the period of focal injury, which can progress to become diffuse through secondary injury mechanisms	• Damage at the cellular/molecular level • Ischemia causes cell death • Vasogenic edema = extracellular edema, associated with cerebral contusion • Cytogenic edema = intracellular edema, associated with hypoxic and ischemic injury

Data from Wagner AK, Arenth PM, Kwasnica C, et al. Traumatic Brain Injury. In: Cifu DX, editor. Braddom's Physical Medicine and Rehabilitation, 5th edition. Philadelphia: Elsevier; 2016; and Elovic E, Baerga E, Galang GF, et al. Traumatic Brain Injury. In: Cuccurullo SJ, editor. Physical Medicine and Rehabilitation Board Review, 2nd edition. New York: Demos Medical Publishing; 2010.

Focal Injury

This type of injury can occur via multiple mechanisms. It is important to understand that, unlike some other neurologic disorders, a focal injury to the brain due to trauma may not produce predictable clinical symptoms.[4] Examples of intracranial pathology resulting from focal injury includes epidural hematoma, subdural hematoma, subarachnoid hemorrhage (in the case of an isolated aneurysm rupture) and intraventricular hemorrhage are presented in **Boxes 2–5**.[2,4]

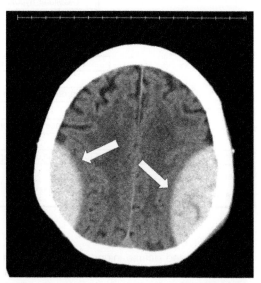

Box 2
Epidural hematoma

• Bleeding outside the dura of the brain (**Fig. 2**)

• Does not cross suture lines

• Classically associated with middle meningeal artery damage

• Clinically may involve a period of loss of consciousness followed by a "lucid" interval with subsequent cognitive decline due to increased intracranial pressure, which can lead to herniation

• Lentiform hyperintensity noted in right (R) frontal region on the left side of the image

Fig. 2. Epidural hematoma (*white arrows*)are pointing at two hyperdense lentiform (lense-shaped or lemon-shaped) areas. In the acute phase, blood appears hyperdense (white) on a CT scan. Epidural hematomas are classically associated with injury to the middle meningeal artery and are considered extradural, as such, they do not typically cross the suture lines of the skull.

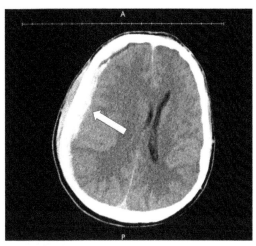

Fig. 3. Subdural hematoma (*white arrow*) is pointing at a crescent shaped hyperdense (white) area demonstrating a subdural hematoma. Subdural hematomas are classically associated with damage to bridging cortical veins and as such they are able to cross suture lines. In this image, you can clearly see compression of the right lateral ventricle and right to left midline shift resulting from the subdural hematoma.

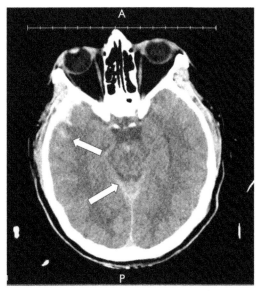

Fig. 4. Subarachnoid hemorrhage. Arrows are pointing to hyperdensities within the subarachnoid space which, in the acute phase, indicates subarachnoid bleeding.

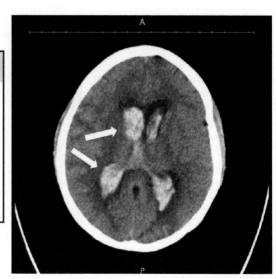

Box 5
Intraventricular hemorrhage

- Bleeding into the ventricles (**Fig. 5**)
- Clinically may be associated with hydrocephalus
- Acute hemorrhage and hydroce-phalus seen by hyperintensity in all ventricles on the left side of the image (arrows)

Fig. 5. Intraventricular hemorrhage. Arrows are pointing to the lateral ventricles of the brain which typically appear hypodense or black on a CT scan. The diffuse hyperdense region within the ventricles demonstrates acute intraventricular hemorrhage.

Diffuse Injury

The presence of diffuse axonal injury on diffusion-weighted imaging studies is associated with a poorer prognosis for recovery.[8] Diffuse injury, as opposed to focal contusion, is associated with disorders of consciousness (DOC) (**Table 6**).

Table 6
Grading of diffuse axonal injury

Grade I	Grade II	Grade III
Affects gray-white matter interface Frontal/ temporal > parietal/occipital	Involves frontal, temporal, parietal, occipital lobes, and corpus callosum	Includes damage to the brainstem as well as damage to structures mentioned in grade I and II

Data from Armstrong M, Chung K, Himmler M, et al. TBI Classifications and Rehabilitation Intensities. In: Eapen BC, Cifu DX, editors. Rehabilitation after Traumatic Brain Injury. St. Louis: Elsevier; 2018.

ACUTE MANAGEMENT
On-Scene Assessment

Following an acute TBI, the patient should be evaluated and medically stabilized as quickly as possible. As in other emergency situations, evaluating the airway, breathing, and circulation is the first step. Problems with circulation, as in a cardiac arrest, may lead to nontraumatic anoxic brain injury.[5]

Acquiring an initial Glasgow Coma Scale (GCS) score will help guide further treatment. It is important to repeat the GCS frequently because mental status can decline in a short period of time, necessitating rapid interventions, such as intubation and transfer to a higher level of care.[5]

Moderate to severe cases of TBI may require intubation and mechanical ventilation for airway protection. Many patients with TBI present with polytrauma. Although other injuries may require emergent attention, the TBI workup should include a prompt complete neurologic examination as well as a computed tomographic (CT) head scan without contrast to evaluate bleeding and CT scan of the cervical spine to evaluate fracture.[5]

Head CT scans are the first-line imaging assessment to reveal an intracranial pathologic condition, which may require surgical intervention. Common intracranial findings include depressed skull fracture, subdural hematoma, epidural hematoma, subarachnoid hemorrhage, and intraventricular hemorrhage. Neurosurgery should be consulted for an intracranial pathologic condition because patients may develop increased pressure inside the brain, causing herniation and death.[5]

A craniotomy is a decompressive surgery in which the skull is replaced immediately. In contrast, a craniectomy is a decompressive surgery in which the bone flap is removed and left off until swelling resolves in the brain and it can be replaced at a later time (replacing the bone is called a cranioplasty). Patients who have a bone flap removed should wear a custom-fitted helmet when upright or out of bed.[5]

Surgeons may place an intracranial pressure (ICP) monitoring device. Examples of this include the extraventricular drain, intraparenchymal catheter, or combination catheter, which allows real-time information about ICP. Neuro–intensive care unit providers often consider additional medical or surgical management once ICP is 20 to 22 mm Hg (normal ICP is 10–15 mm Hg). Practice guidelines exist for ICP management and may involve changing the elevation of the bed, draining CSF, hyperosmolar fluids like mannitol or hypertonic saline (3%), hyperventilation, barbiturate coma, or return to the operating room for further decompression.[5]

Other metrics, such as cerebral perfusion pressure and brain oxygenation, are important in the acute hospitalization phase. Electroencephalogram (EEG) may also be performed to assess sleep/wake cycles and evaluate possible seizure activity.[5]

Although this article focuses on moderate and severe injuries, not all patients who sustain a TBI require advanced head imaging or hospitalization. mTBIs (GCS 13–15) and concussions constitute the vast majority of all TBI cases (80%–90%). The Canadian Computed Tomography Head Rule for Minor Head Injury was developed to help guide clinicians regarding appropriateness of imaging for mTBI and sports-related concussion (**Box 6**).[10]

Post-traumatic Amnesia

Posttraumatic amnesia (PTA) is the period of time between a TBI event and recovery of active memory. Patients in PTA may be ambulating and carrying conversation, but they will be unable to recall details from the conversation soon after. This interval of "lost memory" is one of the most common metrics used to determine severity of injury and prognosis for recovery. PTA is described as retrograde or anterograde. Retrograde amnesia means an inability to retrieve past memories. Anterograde amnesia means an inability to make new memories. For patients with TBI, severe disability is unlikely if PTA lasts less

> **Box 6**
> **Canadian computed tomography head rule for minor head injury**
>
> High risk (for neurologic intervention)
> - Failure to reach 15 on the Glasgow Coma Scale within 2 hours
> - Suspected open skull fracture
> - Any sign of basal skull fracture
> - Two or more vomiting episodes
> - 65 years or older
>
> Medium risk (for brain injury on CT scan)
> - Retrograde amnesia (before impact) more than 30 minutes
> - Dangerous mechanism of injury
>
> *From* Magee DJ. Head and Face. In: Magee DJ, editor. Orthopedic Physical Assessment, 6th edition. St Louis: Saunders; 2014; with permission.

than 2 months. Conversely, functional recovery is unlikely if PTA persists past 3 months.[4]

Several validated tools are available to assess emergence from PTA. These validated tools include the Galveston Orientation and Amnesia Test, the Children's Orientation and Amnesia Test, and The Orientation Log.[2,5,11,12]

MEDICAL MANAGEMENT

Additional medical complications of TBI not discussed in detail within this article include cranial nerve damage, visual disturbances, spatial neglect, balance disorders, and movement disorders.[5]

Posttraumatic Seizures

The International League Against Epilepsy defines seizures as "a transient occurrence of signs and/or symptoms due to abnormal excessive or synchronous neuronal activity in the brain."[13] Posttraumatic seizures are a possible complication of TBI. Seizures following TBI are classified as immediate, early, or late. Focal seizures, formerly known as simple partial (pure motor) seizures, are the most common type to occur late in this population, although others (complex partial, generalized, and so forth) are documented.[7,13] More than 80% of patients who develop seizure activity will present in the first 2 years after injury. Currently, there is no evidence to suggest prolonged prophylaxis with antiepileptic drugs (AEDs) will prevent late seizures.[7] There is evidence that an initial AED loading dose followed by 7 days of AED therapy after an injury can help prevent early seizure. Patients who have documented early seizure activity often will remain on AED therapy for longer than 7 days per Neurosurgery or Neurology recommendations. Although AED therapy may be necessary, sedation is a common side effect that can negatively impact cognition (**Tables 7** and **8**).[5]

Table 7 Posttraumatic seizure classification		
Immediate	Early	Late
<24 h	24 h to 7 d	>7 d

Data from Elovic E, Baerga E, Galang GF, et al. Traumatic Brain Injury. In: Cuccurullo SJ, editor. Physical Medicine and Rehabilitation Board Review, 2nd edition. New York: Demos Medical Publishing; 2010.

Table 8 Incidence of posttraumatic seizure by severity		
Mild	**Moderate**	**Severe**
1.5%	2.9%	17%

Data from Elovic E, Baerga E, Galang GF, et al. Traumatic Brain Injury. In: Cuccurullo SJ, editor. Physical Medicine and Rehabilitation Board Review, 2nd edition. New York: Demos Medical Publishing; 2010.

Posttraumatic Neuroendocrine Disorders

The pituitary gland is sensitive to acceleration and deceleration injuries. Mechanisms of damage include mechanical owing to sella turcica location, interruption of fragile vascular supply, and systemic stress response.[8]

Although neuroendocrine abnormalities are rare in mTBI, hypopituitarism after severe TBI has a prevalence of 50% to 80%. In the acute postinjury phase, hyperprolactinemia was the highest reported complication followed by diabetes insipidus (DI), syndrome of inappropriate adrenocorticotropic hormone (SIADH), human growth hormone (HGH) adrenocorticotropic hormone deficiency (ACTH) deficiency. Addressing these issues can assist both cognitive and physical recovery.[5]

In the absence of clinical suspicion, current guidelines do not suggest routine monitoring of GH, ACTH, thyrotropin, and gonadal axes in the acute phase. It may be helpful to evaluate these hormones in patients with DOC because treatable neuroendocrine disorders may impede emerging consciousness.[5,8]

Posttraumatic Hydrocephalus

Posttraumatic hydrocephalus (PTH) is important to identify because treatment can affect functional outcome. Ventricle enlargement owing to brain tissue atrophy or ex vacuo dilation after craniectomy makes PTH difficult to distinguish on imaging. Considering clinical signs and symptoms is helpful in conjunction with imaging. Treatment will most often involve ventriculoperitoneal shunt placement (**Table 9**).[5]

Table 9 Posttraumatic hydrocephalus	
• Risk factors: Intracranial bleeding, meningitis, postsurgical decompressive craniectomy, coma duration, advanced patient age • Early shunting predicts better outcomes	
Communicating Ventricular system is connected	**Noncommunicating** CSF flow is blocked
CSF flows from ventricles to subarachnoid space This is the most common type seen in TBI Blood products/dead tissue can block flow Often results in normal pressure hydrocephalus Signs/symptoms: 1. Lack of progress/plateau in therapy sessions 2. Ataxia 3. Urinary incontinence 4. Poor initiation 5. Decreased attention 6. Forgetfulness	Signs symptoms: Most are associated with increased ICP 1. Nausea 2. Vomiting 3. Lethargy 4. Headaches 5. Papilledema 6. Gait disturbances

Data from Greenwald BD, Hampton S, Jasey N, et al. Neurologic Complications After Traumatic Brain Injury. In: Eapen BC, Cifu DX, editors. Rehabilitation after Traumatic Brain Injury. St. Louis: Elsevier; 2018; and Wagner AK, Arenth PM, Kwasnica C, et al. Traumatic Brain Injury. In: Cifu DX, editor. Braddom's Physical Medicine and Rehabilitation, 5th edition. Philadelphia: Elsevier; 2016.

Post-traumatic Agitation

Posttraumatic agitation is defined by Braddom's *Physical Medicine and Rehabilitation* as "an excess of one or more behaviors that occurs during an altered state of consciousness." The altered state of consciousness this text alludes to is known as PTA, a common time period during which patients with TBI are unable to form new memories.[2]

Agitation is common in the acute phase after TBI (35%–96% of cases), but can persist long term.[8] Posttraumatic agitation is described as a subset of delirium. Behavioral issues are a major source of morbidity in patients with TBI and cause barriers to reintegration into the home and community. Agitation encompasses behaviors such as irritability, anger, and aggression (verbal or physical). It is important to identify specific behaviors to create a targeted treatment plan.[8]

Common and modifiable risk factors for agitation include an overstimulating environment or unpleasant experience, pain, infection, disrupted sleep patterns, and frontal lobe damage.[5,8]

How to Measure Agitation

Several objective scales exist to track a patient's agitated behaviors. These scales are meant to standardize the way health care providers describe agitation in an effort to provide targeted, successful interventions.

Rancho Los Amigos Scale–Revised

This scale is named for the location where it was developed, an inpatient rehabilitation center in Downey, California. The Rancho scale is meant to describe the typical process of emergence from a coma for patients with severe TBI. This scale is especially helpful for families trying to understand a loved one's recovery (**Table 10**).[14]

Table 10 Rancho Los Amigos Scale–revised		
Level	**Clinical Examination**	**Functional Independence Measure**
I	No response	Total assist
II	Generalized response	Total assist
III	Localized response	Total assist
IV	Confused and agitated	Maximal assist
V	Confused and inappropriate, nonagitated	Maximal assist
VI	Confused and appropriate	Moderate assist
VII	Automatic and appropriate	Minimal assist
VIII	Purposeful, appropriate	Stand-by assist
IX	Purposeful, appropriate	Stand-by assist
X	Purposeful, appropriate	Modified independence

Adapted from Centre for Neuro Skills (CNS). Rancho Los Amigos Scale – Revised. Available at: https://www.neuroskills.com/education-and-resources/rancho-los-amigos-revised/. Accessed Oct 18 2019; with permission.

Common Neuropsychiatric Disorders Following Traumatic Brain Injury

General rules to successfully interact with a patient after acute TBI (**Table 11**) include[2] the following:

1. *Patients may be easily confused and have impaired memory:* Reorient the patient frequently. Use simple language. When providing an explanation, try to avoid giving

Table 11 Neuropsychiatric disorders: common chronic complications associated with traumatic brain injury	
Major depression	• Most common mood disorder associated with TBI • Prevalence range 6% to 90% • Premorbid depression associated with depression postinjury
Anxiety	• Second most common disorder behind depression • Associated with cognitive fatigue • Selective serotonin reuptake inhibitors (SSRIs) can be effective in patients with TBI
Posttraumatic stress disorder	• Increased severity of injury may be protective against this • Patients with TBI do not need to recall the event to develop this condition
Psychosis	• Ensure not caused by medication side effects (amantadine) • Can be well managed with atypical antipsychotics • Avoid typical antipsychotics caused by dopamine-depleting properties
Paranoia	• Associated with PTA • Commonly persists long term after TBI • Reports of success with atypical antipsychotics
Pseudobulbar affect	• Characterized by inappropriate emotional response, such as random outbursts of laughing/crying • Treatment options include dextromethorphan HBr and quinidine sulfate, SSRIs, tricyclic antidepressants (TCAs)
Aggression	• Associated with emergence from PTA but can present at any time after TBI • Multimodal management with behavioral, environmental, and medication strategies • Beta-blockers, mood stabilizers, SSRIs, and atypical antipsychotics are medications most often used

Data from Ripley DL, Driver S, Stork R, et al. Pharmacologic Management of the Patient With Traumatic Brain Injury. In: Eapen BC, Cifu DX, editors. Rehabilitation after Traumatic Brain Injury. St. Louis: Elsevier; 2018.

too much information all at once (1 concept at a time). Allow extra time for explanations. Patients may be disinhibited and come across as rude; do not take this behavior personally.[2]

2. *Overstimulation can lead to irritable or agitated behavior; instead, provide a low stimulation environment:* Limit distractions and noise in the room (ie, turn off the radio or television, dim the lights, limit the number of people in the room to one or two, only allow 1 person to talk at a time). When giving instructions, provide simple step-by-step directions; depending on the patient's cognitive function, it may be appropriate to provide a written copy. Redirect patients when they become frustrated with an activity; allow rest breaks as needed. Consider that a patient may be experiencing pain or fatigue and may have trouble expressing this. Consider addressing these underlying issues to help improve their behavior.[2]

3. *Patients with TBI may be impulsive and lack safety awareness:* When addressing a patient, get their attention before you speak. Approach a patient slowly and always from the front, not from behind. Speak slowly, clearly, and softly. Use the patient's name frequently in conversation. Use demonstration, not just verbal instruction, and provide written material if relevant.[2]

First-Line Treatment for an Agitated Patient: Behavioral Interventions

Because of impaired cognition and communication, patients with TBI often have a hard time expressing an underlying problem, which can then manifest as agitated behavior. Consider possible medical reasons for agitation. Common medical triggers for agitation include urinary tract infection, respiratory infection, constipation, urinary retention, pain, and dehydration. It is reasonable to consider a basic workup for infection, including a urinalysis, a metabolic panel, and a complete blood count, to assess electrolytes and inflammatory markers. Occasionally, patients experience posttraumatic hydrocephalus or shunt malfunction if a shunt was previously placed, and obtaining a CT head scan without contrast may be reasonable depending on the case and presentation.[2]

Once medical causes for agitation are ruled out or treated, nonpharmacologic interventions are considered first line in behavioral management. Address overstimulation as described earlier, and providing a low stimulation environment is often a key for an agitated patient. Ensure the patient is protected from harming themselves and other people. Tolerate restlessness when possible because physically restraining a patient often leads to more anxiety and agitated behaviors. Interventions, such as using a floor bed with side panels, having a 1:1 sitter, video monitoring, and use of a locked ward, may be helpful. Restraints should only be used when absolutely necessary. If needed, consider using unrestrained hand mittens to prevent pulling at lines/tubes rather than wrist and ankle restraints. If able, keep health care providers consistent so the patient is able to see familiar faces daily.[2]

Pharmacologic Agitation Management

There is little evidence to support or refute use of medications for agitation in TBI based on the current literature (**Tables 12** and **13**).[15] The following is a list of mood stabilizers commonly used for agitation management.

Table 12 Pharmacologic management of agitation	
Medication Class	**Examples**
Nonspecific beta-blockers	Propranolol, pindolol, metoprolol
Neuro stimulants	Methylphenidate, modafinil, amantadine, donepezil
Antipsychotics	Olanzapine, quetiapine, risperidone
SSRIs	Fluoxetine, sertraline
Anticonvulsants	Valproic acid, carbamazepine
TCAs	Amitriptyline, nortriptyline, desipramine
Benzodiazepines	Diazepam, lorazepam
Norepinephrine and dopamine reuptake inhibitors	Buspirone
Alpha-2-agonist	Clonidine
Opiates[a]	Morphine, oxycodone, and similar

[a] If pain is triggering agitation.

Data from Ripley DL, Driver S, Stork R, et al. Pharmacologic Management of the Patient With Traumatic Brain Injury. In: Eapen BC, Cifu DX, editors. Rehabilitation after Traumatic Brain Injury. St. Louis: Elsevier; 2018.

Table 13
Dopamine-promoting agents may assist in cognitive recovery after severe traumatic brain injury

Medication	Mechanism of Action	Common Side Effects
Methylphenidate	Amphetamine	Tachycardia
Amantadine	Dopamine agonist	Lowers seizure threshold Orthostatic hypotension Visual hallucinations
Levodopa/Carbidopa	Dopamine agonist	Orthostatic hypotension, dizziness, nausea, Headache (HA)
Bromocriptine	Dopamine agonist	Nausea, HA, Dizziness
Donepezil (adults)	Acetylcholinesterase inhibitor	Insomnia

Data from Neurobehavioral Guidelines Working Group, Warden DL, Gordon B, et al. Guidelines for the Pharmacologic Treatment of Neurobehavioral Sequelae of Traumatic Brain Injury. J Neurotrauma 2006;23(10):1468-1501.

Carbamazepine

Mechanism of Action: Activates K+ channels, Na channel blocker, regulates limbic kindling
Common side effects: Aplastic anemia, hyponatremia, ataxia, nausea, agranulocytosis, sedation, toxic epidermal necrolysis[5,16]
Food and Drug Administration (FDA) indications: Trigeminal neuralgia, seizures

Lamotrigine

Mechanism of Action: Glutamate antagonist, inhibits Na channels
Common side effects: Headache, dizziness, diplopia, toxic epidermal necrolysis, fatigue

Valproic acid

Mechanism of Action: Delays repolarization of Na channels, increases GABA activity, controls limbic kindling, NMDA antagonist
Common side effects: Hepatotoxicity, somnolence, thrombocytopenia, weight gain
FDA indications: Neuropathic pain, alcohol withdrawal
In a randomized controlled trial, this drug did not demonstrate damage to cognition.

What to avoid and why

When treating a patient with TBI with behavioral disorders, avoid dopamine antagonist medications when able. Current literature suggests these medications may prolong PTA and inhibit cognitive recovery. Haloperidol, a commonly used medication for agitation, is a dopamine antagonist. Alternatives, including olanzapine and risperidone, likely have a similar risk, and there are studies with conflicting results, although data are difficult to interpret because of small population sizes. Medications commonly used to treat behavioral disorders after TBI can be associated with side effects (**Table 14**).

Table 14
Common adverse effects reported in patients with traumatic brain injury with standard pharmacologic interventions

Beta-Blockers	Hypotension, bradycardia, fatigue
TCAs	Seizures
Clozapine	Weight gain, drooling, seizures
Desipramine	Mania
Fluoxetine	Dysarthria, aphasia
Sertraline	Akathisia
Paroxetine	Akathisia
Lithium	Cognitive impairments, narrow therapeutic index, neurotoxicity

Although these medications can help in certain instances, impaired cognition may be a side effect due to the ability to cross the blood brain barrier resulting in sedation.[5]

Data from Neurobehavioral Guidelines Working Group, Warden DL, Gordon B, et al. Guidelines for the Pharmacologic Treatment of Neurobehavioral Sequelae of Traumatic Brain Injury. J Neurotrauma 2006;23(10):1468-1501.

Agitated Behavior Scale

This instrument was published in 1995. The goal of the Agitated Behavior Scale is to assess patients with agitation after an acute acquired brain injury, such as TBI. The tool is meant to allow frequent documentation for behaviors to help providers identify a trigger or temporal relationship to agitation. The Overt Agitation Severity Scale (not specific to TBI) and the Neurobehavioral Rating Scale (monitors agitation and PTA) are 2 additional tools developed more recently.[2]

Paroxysmal Sympathetic Hyperactivity ("Storming")

After a brain injury, patients may experience paroxysmal sympathetic hyperactivity. Common synonyms used include paroxysmal autonomic instability and dystonia syndrome and "storming." A hyperadrenergic state leading to posttraumatic agitation is the underlying theory behind this process. Storming features are seen in multiple types of acquired brain injuries, including traumatic, anoxic, and stroke,[17,18] and include the following:

- Occurs in 15% to 33% of patients with severe TBI (GCS <8)
- Typical time course: 24 hours to weeks after injury
- Signs: Tachycardia, hyperthermia, dystonia, posturing, diaphoresis, hypertension, pupillary dilatation, tachypnea
- Common mimics: Neuroleptic malignant syndrome, serotonin syndrome, sepsis
- Common triggers: Infection, pain, overstimulation, constipation, urinary retention, insomnia
- Nonpharmacologic treatments: Repositioning, massage, cool cloths, soothing music
- Pharmacologic treatments: Propranolol, clonidine, bromocriptine, gabapentin

Spasticity

Spasticity is defined as a velocity-dependent, involuntary resistance to a passive stretch. It is a known complication of moderate to severe TBI. The mechanism is attributed to central injuries, which cause loss of inhibitory signals, impairing the normal stretch reflex. The result is an increase in muscle tone, which can be painful and impaired motor function and range of motion. However, tone may be used functionally to help patients transfer or walk, in some cases; this principle becomes important when developing a treatment plan. Spasticity is not isolated to TBI and is seen in several neurologic disorders.[5]

Spasticity management requires a multimodal approach. Initial management includes range-of-motion exercises, stretching, splinting, and bracing. Oral medications, focal injections, and intrathecal baclofen pump placement are other options. Although oral medications are often trialed first for spasticity, nearly all are sedating, which can impair cognition and overall function. Focal injections with botulinum toxin or phenol may be performed for targeted areas, depending on functional goals. Tone can impair ambulation as well as the ability to dress, transfer, and perform hygiene.[5]

Spasticity can be a symptom of an underlying noxious stimulus (such as a full bladder, constipation, infection, or a pressure wound). If spasticity becomes markedly worse without explanation, it is reasonable to evaluate the patient for an underlying trigger (**Table 15**).

Table 15
Pharmacology of spasticity management

Commonly Used Medications for Spasticity Management		
Medication	Mechanism of Action	Side Effects and Special Considerations
Baclofen (oral)	Centrally acting GABA analogue that binds to GABA-B receptors to inhibit muscle stretch reflex and decrease motor neuron activity at the spinal cord level	Somnolence, fatigue, muscle weakness, xerostomia, urinary retention, constipation, elevated liver function tests (LFTs) Abrupt cessation is associated with withdrawal, including altered mental status, hallucinations, seizures, increased muscle tone, and spasms
Baclofen (intrathecal)	Same as above	Reduced systemic side effects when compared with oral because intrathecal delivery allows for higher concentration at a lower dose Withdrawal symptoms are related to a malfunction with the baclofen pump device or damage to the catheter
Tizanidine	Alpha-2 agonist that inhibits the release of excitatory neurotransmitters (glutamate, aspartate) from spinal interneurons	Somnolence, dizziness, hypotension, xerostomia, elevated LFTs
Dantrolene	Inhibits the release of calcium from the sarcoplasmic reticulum of muscle, interfering with skeletal muscle contraction	Muscle weakness, drowsiness, diarrhea, hepatotoxicity; often preferred for TBI-induced spasticity because it acts peripherally
Gabapentin	GABA analogue, although mechanism of action is not well understood	Drowsiness, dizziness, edema

(continued on next page)

	Table 15 (continued)	
	Commonly Used Medications for Spasticity Management	
Medication	**Mechanism of Action**	**Side Effects and Special Considerations**
Diazepam	Binds to GABA-A receptor, facilitating chloride influx and inducing neuronal inhibition	Sedation, cognitive impairments; abrupt cessation can lead to withdrawal symptoms
Clonidine	Centrally acting alpha-2 agonist that decreases sympathetic outflow	Hypotension, rebound hypertension, bradycardia, xerostomia, drowsiness, constipation, depression
Botulinum toxin	Inhibits presynaptic acetylcholine release by cleaving the SNAP-25 protein in the SNARE complex	Weakness, fatigue, flulike symptoms, dysphagia, complications associated with the procedure, such as infection, bleeding, and pain; short-term effect (3–6 mo)
Phenol	Neurotoxin that denatures proteins in the area surrounding the injection site	Dysesthesias, hypotension, prolonged pain, complications associated with procedure, such as infection, bleeding, and pain Longer lasting than botulinum toxin (6 mo to 1 y)

Adapted from Eapen BC, Hong S, Subbarao B, et al. Medical Complications After Moderate to Severe Traumatic Brain Injury. In: Eapen BC, Cifu DX, editors. Rehabilitation after Traumatic Brain Injury. St. Louis: Elsevier; 2018; with permission.

Heterotopic ossification

Heterotopic ossification (HO) is a phenomenon seen in several neurologic and orthopedic injuries. Lamellar bone forms in soft tissue and can severely limit a joint's range of motion and function. The mechanism is poorly understood. The frequency of occurrence has a wide range with reports as low as 4% and as high as 23%. In patients with TBI, the hips, knees, and shoulders are the most common areas of HO formation. HO is challenging to detect. The presentation is often similar to a bone fracture, septic joint, cellulitis, or deep venous thrombosis (DVT). Laboratory workup with inflammatory markers is nonspecific. Diagnostic tools include bone scans and ultrasound, although these are also nonspecific. Radiographs will not show HO until it is advanced, making treatment difficult. Treatment options include nonsteroidal anti-inflammatory drugs, bisphosphonates, and radiation therapy in the early stages and surgical resection in the later stages. Despite treatment, HO often recurs.[5]

Hypercoagulability

Patients with moderate to severe TBI requiring hospitalization and subsequent immobilization are at increased risk for DVT and pulmonary embolism. In the absence of any prevention measures, 20% to 25% of patients with TBI develop a DVT. However, many hospitalized patients with TBI have evidence of recent intracranial bleeding, and thus, the benefit of chemoprophylaxis must be weighed against the possibility of bleeding. No clear guidelines exist to determine timing of starting chemoprophylaxis.[5]

Malnutrition

Patients with TBI, particularly those with severe injuries, have increased caloric needs following injury. These metabolic changes are attributed to an inflammatory state.

Although TBI is associated with a 75% to 200% increase in energy expenditure, the use of sedatives and presence of disorders of consciousness (DOC) decrease metabolism. Because many hospitalized patients with TBI are unable to eat orally, it is important to start enteral feeding as soon as possible with a focus on delivering a high-protein diet (2–2.5 g/kg/d). There is evidence to suggest early feeding (within 48 hours) can decrease neuroendocrine complications.[5]

CONCUSSION

Concussion has been used synonymously with the term mTBI. Emerging classification mechanisms specific to concussion promote separation of these terms. Mild injuries likely account for more than 80% of all TBI, although the true incidence is difficult to ascertain because many patients who sustain these injuries do not seek medical attention, and therefore, they are not documented or tracked. Most research and subsequent assessment tools are focused on sports-related concussion.[19]

The 2017 fifth edition of the Standardized Concussion Assessment Tool is validated for patients 13 years and older; a child version exists for younger patients. This tool is a comprehensive evaluation and includes orientation questions, a GCS, a neurologic screen, a cervical spine test, a cognitive screen, balance testing, and a symptom checklist. Several other postconcussion patient self-assessment tools are available for patients experiencing persistent symptoms.[19]

When evaluating a patient after a concussion, consider these important red-flag features, which may warrant further workup and imaging. Red-flag signs include loss of consciousness greater than 30 seconds, posttraumatic amnesia greater than 30 minutes, seizure activity, vomiting, severe headache, focal neurologic findings, and limited or painful neck range of motion.

The vast majority of patients with mTBI will recover within 1 to 2 weeks. Current literature suggests up to 15% of patients will experience persistent postconcussive symptoms, although the term "postconcussion syndrome" is typically reserved for patients with multiple symptom complaints that persist for many months to years after their injury.[20] Although the mechanism for development of postconcussion syndrome is not well understood, several factors, including social, biological, and psychological, likely play a role. Linking symptoms directly to mTBI can be challenging because the associated symptoms are common in the general population. Postconcussion headache is the most common symptom. Other symptoms include sleep dysfunction, cognitive dysfunction, vestibular disorders, visual/spatial dysfunction, irritability, and emotional lability.[19,20]

DISORDERS OF CONSCIOUSNESS (DISTURBANCES OF CONSCIOUSNESS)

Consciousness is a function of the ascending reticular activating system and the cerebral cortex. The term DOC describes a state of prolonged altered consciousness, which is categorized into coma, vegetative state (VS), and minimally conscious state (MCS) depending on the presence of arousal and awareness of self and environment (**Table 16**).[21]

Table 16 Disorders of consciousness			
	Coma	VS (Unresponsive Wakefulness Syndrome)	MCS
Arousal	Absent	Present	Present
Awareness	Absent	Absent	Present

Data from Giacino JT, Fins JJ, Laureys S, et al. Disorders of consciousness after acquired brain injury: the state of the science. Nat Rev Neurol 2014;10(2):99-114.

A coma is a state of unconsciousness with no evidence of arousal and awareness. There is no eye-opening or sleep-wake cycle on EEG. Those who survive this state will transition to either VS or minimally conscious state (MCS) within 2 to 4 weeks.

A VS, also known as unresponsive wakefulness syndrome, reflects the dissociation between wakefulness and awareness. In a VS, sleep-wake cycles are evident on EEG. Patients may arouse with external stimuli as demonstrated by intermittent eye opening, but they do not show signs of perception or purposeful movement. Patients in VS may show stereotyped gestural movements, such as yawning, chewing, auditory/visual startle, vocalization, crying, smiling, and moaning without contingence, but they do not indicate the presence of awareness.[22]

An MCS is characterized by a severe impairment of consciousness with evidence of wakefulness and preservation of awareness. Awareness refers to the ability of an individual to respond to both external and internal stimuli. These patients can demonstrate inconsistent, but reproducible command following, nonreflexive movement, object manipulation, localization of pain, visual pursuit, verbalization, contingent affective response, and so forth.[5]

One is considered to have emerged from MCS (eMCS) once he or she performs *functional* object use (eg, bringing a cup to his or her mouth) or *functional interactive* communication (eg, accurate response to yes or no questions).[22]

Assessment and Diagnosis

Correctly determining the level of consciousness for DOC patients is often challenging, especially when confounding factors, such as sensory, motor, and cognitive impairments that mimic DOC, are present (**Box 7**). Also, it is important to address and treat reversible causes for impaired consciousness, such as sedating medications, concurrent medical issues, and unrecognized intracranial abnormalities before the assessment (**Box 8**). Making a correct diagnosis is important for several reasons. Access to specialized rehabilitation services is much more limited for individuals thought to be in VS than for someone in MCS. Rehabilitation goals also differ based on the perceived level of consciousness (eg, enhancing arousal for VS vs establishing a communication system for MCS).

Box 7
Examples of mimics and confounding factors of disorders of consciousness

Mimics
- Locked-in syndrome
- Catatonia
- Akinetic mutism

Confounding factors
- Widespread paresis or paralysis (eg, critical illness myopathy, critical illness neuropathy)
- Profound sensory deficits (eg, blindness, deafness)
- Bilateral cranial nerve III palsy
- Diffuse spasticity and contracture
- High-order cognitive deficits (eg, aphasia, apraxia)

Adapted from Kothari S, Gilbert-Baffoe E, O'Brien KA. Disorders of Consciousness. In: Eapen BC, Cifu DX, editors. Rehabilitation after Traumatic Brain Injury. St. Louis: Elsevier; 2018; with permission.

Box 8
Reversible causes of impaired consciousness

- Seizures (eg, subclinical seizure, nonconvulsive status epilepticus)
- Neuroendocrine abnormalities (eg, growth hormone deficiency, thyroid function abnormalities)
- Infection (eg, urinary tract infection, pneumonia, meningitis)
- Metabolic abnormalities (eg, hyponatremia, hypoglycemia)
- Intracranial abnormalities (eg, hydrocephalus, progressive intracranial bleed)
- Sedating medication (eg, anticholinergic, GABAergic, antidopaminergic)
- Disrupted sleep-wake cycle

Adapted from Kothari S, Gilbert-Baffoe E, O'Brien KA. Disorders of Consciousness. In: Eapen BC, Cifu DX, editors. Rehabilitation after Traumatic Brain Injury. St. Louis: Elsevier; 2018; with permission.

Although bedside evaluation can help diagnose a patient's level of consciousness, these subjective evaluations need to be supplemented by formal assessments because observed responses are often subtle. One study discovered 41% of patients diagnosed with VS based on the clinical consensus were actually in an MCS following standardized behavioral assessment (see later discussion).[23]

Clinicians should keep in mind that the level of consciousness may continue to fluctuate during recovery and can yield inconsistent behaviors. For that reason, formal evaluations should be performed multiple times with different modes of assessment by multiple examiners at various times of day under optimal environmental conditions.[5]

In general, behavioral assessments are considered the "gold standard" for determining the presence and level of consciousness. Specialists use the Coma Recovery Scale Revised and/or the Individualized Quantitative Behavioral Assessment, which are comprehensive scales useful in detecting subtle presence or changes in consciousness. Nonbehavioral assessments are performed using various diagnostic tools, such as pupillometry, surface electromyography, functional MRI scan, and transcranial magnetic stimulation coupled with EEG, to detect consciousness that is not behaviorally evident. It is important to note that there is a high rate of false negative results with nonbehavioral assessments. Negative responses should not be used to exclude the possible presence of consciousness.[5]

Treatment

Once reversible causes and confounding factors are identified and addressed, interventions to enhance the level of consciousness should be considered. Consciousness assessments should continue during this phase as patients may transition to different states (eg, VS to MCS, MCS to eMCS). Treatment modalities can be divided into pharmacologic and nonpharmacologic categories as listed in **Box 9**.[5]

Applied energy therapy modalities, such as transcranial direct current stimulation (tDCS), repetitive transcranial magnetic stimulation (rTMS), deep brain stimulation (DBS), and right median nerve stimulation, are currently being investigated. In order

---

Box 9
Interventions to enhance the level of consciousness

Pharmacologic Treatment	Nonpharmacologic Treatment
Hypoarousal	Mobilization
• Amantadine	• Sitting program
• Bromocriptine	• Standing program
• Modafinil	• Body-weight-supported therapeutic gait
• Levodopa	
• Zolpidem	Sensory stimulation
	• Tactile, auditory, visual, vestibular, and
Attention/processing speed	Interpersonal interaction
• Methylphenidate	
• Dextroamphetamine	Applied energy therapy
	• tDCS
Memory	• rTMS
• Donepezil	• DBS
• Memantine	• Right median nerve stimulation

Modified from Kothari S, Gilbert-Baffoe E, O'Brien KA. Disorders of Consciousness. In: Eapen BC, Cifu DX, editors. Rehabilitation after Traumatic Brain Injury. St. Louis: Elsevier; 2018; with permission.

---

to provide accurate diagnostic evaluation, prognostication, and subsequent management, the new American Academy of Neurology guidelines recommend that clinicians should refer DOC patients to multidisciplinary rehabilitation teams whereby the patients will be treated with the goals listed in **Box 10**.[24]

Box 10
Goals of a disorders-of-consciousness program

- Assess current level of consciousness
- Address reversible causes of impaired consciousness
- Initiate interventions to enhance consciousness
- Establish a system of communication
- Identify and magnify residual voluntary movement
- Address restrictions in range of motion
- Intensive mobilization and environmental enrichment
- Prevent and manage secondary medical complications
- Optimize respiration/nutrition/elimination/integument
- Provide family education/training/support
- Establish a plan for aftercare

From Kothari S, Gilbert-Baffoe E, O'Brien KA. Disorders of Consciousness. In: Eapen BC, Cifu DX, editors. Rehabilitation After Traumatic Brain Injury. St. Louis: Elsevier; 2018; with permission.

Prognosis and Outcomes in Disorders of Consciousness

In general, patients in MCS have a more favorable prognosis than those in VS.[25] Within the VS group, traumatic cause carries a better prognosis than nontraumatic cause.[26]

Recent studies show long-term recovery is possible beyond 1 year after injury. One study found that approximately 20% of patients in traumatic VS admitted to a comprehensive inpatient rehabilitation program were functionally independent and capable of returning to employment at 1, 2, or 5 years.[27] Another study noted 88% to 100% of people who regained command-following within 28 days after injury and 50% to 75% of patients who did not were independent on the cognitive, mobility, and self-care functional independence measure scores by 10 years.[28] These findings suggest individuals with DOC may continue to benefit from ongoing functional monitoring and care plans for years after injury.

Ethical Considerations in Disorders of Consciousness

In the United States, individuals on mechanical ventilation with a GCS score of 5 or less are considered for organ procurement.[29] In-hospital mortality for patients with severe TBI (including DOC) is as high as 32%, with 70% of those deaths associated with withdrawal of life-sustaining therapy.[30] Given the diagnostic and prognostic uncertainty in DOC, health care providers may be at risk of starting discussions about limiting or withdrawing medical treatments prematurely while the patients may have the potential to recover, or have already recovered, consciousness. Another common ethical issue arises from patients' limited ability to consent for medical treatment, procedures, and research. In any ethically complicated situations, consulting an ethics committee is recommended.

SOCIAL CONSIDERATIONS
Disposition for Patients After Traumatic Brain Injury

Several options exist for rehabilitation services following acute hospitalization. The level of rehabilitation depends on several factors, including the patients' functional deficits, rehabilitation goals, and therapy participation. Current literature demonstrates improved outcomes for patients who complete an intensive rehabilitation program after TBI. High-quality evidence suggests patients with severe TBI who complete intensive inpatient rehabilitation in an inpatient rehabilitation facility (IRF) demonstrate earlier gains in independence, reduced length of acute hospital stay, and substantial cost savings.[5,8]

IRFs offer a resource-intensive program completed in a hospital setting. Patients must have nursing, medical, and rehabilitation needs that necessitate this level of care. They must require at least 2 therapy subspecialties (between physical therapy, occupational therapy, and speech therapy). In addition, they should be willing and able to participate in 3 or more hours of therapy per day, 5 out of 7 days per week. Physiatrists are generally the primary providers for patients at IRFs. Physiatrists manage rehabilitation-related medical needs, evaluate splinting and bracing needs, and oversee therapy services and durable medical equipment ordering with the goal of maximizing patient function. Interdisciplinary rounds are held once per week on each patient involving the physical, occupational, and speech therapists, physicians, nurses, and other staff members, which may include a neuropsychologist, recreational therapist, dietician, social worker, and case manager. These rounds are tailored to addressing the patient's progress toward functional goals, assessing barriers, and determining an appropriate discharge plan.[31]

For medically complicated patients unable to tolerate 3 hours of therapy per day, a long-term acute care hospital (LTACH) may be appropriate. LTACH patients receive about 1 hour of therapy per day, 5 days per week, and are still seen daily by a physician.[5,31]

Subacute rehabilitation in a skilled nursing facility (SNF) may be an option for patients who do not qualify for acute inpatient rehabilitation at an IRF, but are unable to discharge home. SNF patients are typically more medically stable than those in LTACHs. SNFs and LTACH facilities offer regular therapy services, generally including physical, occupational, and speech therapy. The rigor of therapy will vary, but patients typically receive 5 hours of therapy per week in these centers.[5,31]

If a patient is medically stable enough to discharge home, they have a capable care-giver, and/or they are physically able to navigate their home environment, outpatient therapy may be an option after hospital discharge. Outpatient therapy services in a clinic familiar with neurologic injuries can offer high-quality rehabilitation.[5,31]

Home health services are an option for home-bound medically stable patients not requiring acute or subacute level rehabilitation. Home health services may include a comprehensive home-safety evaluation as well as nursing care, physical, occupational and speech therapies.[5,8]

Primary Prevention

In the 1990s, the Federal Government noticed the rising incidence of TBI and TBI-related disability in the United States. Several programs were enacted through the CDC in an effort to track TBI outcomes, promote brain injury awareness, and identify ways to prevent TBI.[32] At that time, MVC was the number one mechanism of injury. A decrease in MVC as the mechanism of injury is attributed to improved motor vehicle safety features. Growing use of these features, including seatbelts, airbags, car seats, motorcycle helmets as well as improved driver's safety standards, are attributed to a decrease in MVC-related TBI. Although sports helmets do not appear to prevent concussion, they are attributed to preventing more severe injuries.[33] In addition, growing concussion awareness in sports may help identify TBIs earlier, and treating them appropriately may improve long-term morbidity and mortality.[32,33]

SUMMARY

TBI is a prevalent condition in the United States. This prevalence highlights the need for increased awareness of the unique characteristics of this population across medical specialties. Patients with TBI are often misunderstood and misdiagnosed, particularly in the DOC population whereby several confounding factors may be at play. Although PM&R brain injury specialists are important in addressing the sequelae of TBI, an interdisciplinary approach is essential to patients' success considering the medical, surgical, and psychological effects of this diagnosis.

DISCLOSURE

The authors have nothing to disclose.

REFERENCES

1. Surveillance Report of Traumatic Brain Injury-related Emergency Department Visits, Hospitalizations, and Deaths. In: Centers for Disease Control and Prevention, U.S. Department of Health and Human Services. 2014. Available at: https://www.cdc.gov/traumaticbraininjury/get_the_facts.html. Accessed July 8, 2019.
2. Cifu D. Traumatic brain injury. In: Cifu DX, editor. Braddom's physical medicine & rehabilitation. 5th edition. Philadelphia: Elsevier, Inc.; 2016. p. 964, 974, 979–80, 984–8.
3. Jackson G, Hamilton N, Tupler L. Detecting traumatic brain injury among veterans of Operations Enduring and Iraqi Freedom. N C Med J 2008;69:43–7.

4. Zasler ND, Katz DI, Zafonte RD. Brain injury medicine. 2nd edition. New York: Demos Medical Publishing, LLC; 2013.

5. Eapen B, Cifu D. Rehabilitation after traumatic brain injury. St. Louis (MO): Elsevier Inc.; 2018.

6. National database: 2017 profile of people within the traumatic brain injury model systems. Traumatic brain injury model systems National Data and Statistical Center. Center. Available at: https://msktc.org/lib/docs/Data_Sheets_/2017_TBIMS_National_Database_Update_1.pdf. Accessed July 18, 2019.

7. Cuccurullo SJ. Traumatic brain injury. In: Cuccurullo SJ, editor. Physical medicine and rehabilitation board review. 2nd edition. New York: demosMedical; 2010. p. 49–50, 51-3, 90-1.

8. Oberholzer M, Muri R. Neurorehabilitation of traumatic brain injury (TBI): a clinical review. Med Sci 2019;7:1–17.

9. Dixon K. Pathophysiology of traumatic brain injury. Phys Med Rehabil Clin N Am 2017;28:215–25.

10. Magee DJ. Chapter 2, head and face. In: Orthopedic physical assessment. St Louis (MO): Elsevier Saunders; 2014. p. 84–147.

11. Levin HS, O'Donnell VM, Grossman RG. The Galveston Orientation and Amnesia Test: a practical scale to assess cognition after head injury. J Nerv Ment Dis 1979; 167:675–84.

12. Novack T, Dowler R, Bush B, et al. Validity of the orientation log relative to the Galveston Orientation and Amnesia Test. J Head Trauma Rehabil 2000;15:957–61.

13. Berg AT, Berkovic SF, Brodie MJ, et al. Revised terminology and concepts for organization of seizures and epilepsies: report of the ILAE Commission on Classification and Terminology, 2005–2009. Epilepsia 2010;51:676–85.

14. The Rancho Los Amigos scale–revised. Available at: https://www.neuroskills.com/education-and-resources/rancho-los-amigos-revised/. Accessed July 12, 2019.

15. Warden D, Gordon B, McAllister T, et al. Guidelines for the pharmacologic treatment of neurobehavioral sequelae of traumatic brain injury. J Neurotrauma 2006; 23:1468–501.

16. Kalra I, Watanabe T. Mood stabilizers for traumatic brain injury-related agitation. J Head Trauma Rehabil 2017;32:E61–4.

17. Compton E. Paroxysmal sympathetic hyperactivity syndrome following traumatic brain injury. Nurs Clin North Am 2018;53:457–67.

18. Kapoor D, Singla D, Singh J, et al. Paroxysmal autonomic instability with dystonia (PAID) syndrome following cardiac arrest. Singapore Med J 2014;55:123–5.

19. McCrea MA, Nelson LD, Guskiewicz K. Diagnosis and management of acute concussion. Phys Med Rehabil Clin N Am 2017;28:271–86.

20. Tapia RN, Eapen BC. Rehabilitation of persistent symptoms after concussion. Phys Med Rehabil Clin N Am 2017;28:287–99.

21. Eapen BC, Georgekutty J, Subbarao B, et al. Disorders of consciousness. Phys Med Rehabil Clin N Am 2017;28(2):245–58.

22. Giacino JT, Fins JJ, Laureys S, et al. Disorders of consciousness after acquired brain injury: the state of the science. Nat Rev Neurol 2014;10(2):99–114.

23. Schnakers C, Vanhaudenhuyse A, Giacino J, et al. Diagnostic accuracy of the vegetative and minimally conscious state: clinical consensus versus standardized neurobehavioral assessment. BMC Neurol 2009;9:35.

24. Giacino JT, Katz DI, Schiff ND, et al. Practice guideline update recommendations summary: disorders of consciousness. Neurology 2018;91(10):450–60.

25. Giacino JT. The vegetative and minimally conscious states: consensus-based criteria for establishing diagnosis and prognosis. NeuroRehabilitation 2004; 19(4):293–8.

26. The Multi-Society Task Force on PVS. Medical aspects of the persistent vegetative state. N Engl J Med 1994;330:1499–508.

27. Nakase-Richardson R, Whyte J, Giacino JT, et al. Longitudinal outcome of patients with disordered consciousness in the NIDRR TBI model systems programs. J Neurotrauma 2012;29(1):59–65.

28. Hammond FM, Giacino JT, Richardson RN, et al. Disorders of consciousness due to traumatic brain injury: functional status ten years post-injury. J Neurotrauma 2019;36(7):1136–46.

29. Fins JJ. Severe brain injury and organ solicitation: a call for temperance. AMA J Ethics 2012;14(3):221–6.

30. Turgeon AF, Lauzier F, Simard J-F, et al. Mortality associated with withdrawal of life-sustaining therapy for patients with severe traumatic brain injury: a Canadian multicentre cohort study. Can Med Assoc J 2011;183(14):1581–8.

31. Chapter 1–Inpatient hospital services covered under part A. In: Medicare benefit policy manual. 2017. Available at: https://www.cms.gov/Regulations-and-Guidance/Guidance/Manuals/Downloads/bp102c01.pdf. Accessed July 9, 2019.

32. Coronado V, McGuire L, Sarmiento K, et al. Trends in traumatic brain injury in the U.S. and the public health response: 1995-2009. J Safety Res 2012;43: 299–307.

33. Benson BW, Hamilson GM, Meeuwisse WH, et al. Is protective equipment useful in preventing concussion? A systematic review of the literature. Br J Sports Med 2009;43:56–67.

Cancer Rehabilitation

Acute and Chronic Issues, Nerve Injury, Radiation Sequelae, Surgical and Chemo-Related, Part 1

Cristina Kline-Quiroz, DO[a], Phalgun Nori, MD[b],
Michael D. Stubblefield, MD[c],*

KEYWORDS

- Cancer • Rehabilitation • Disability • Function • Quality of life • Neuropathy
- Radiation fibrosis syndrome • Survivorship

KEY POINTS

- Individuals with cancer commonly experience functional impairments.
- Symptoms may present immediately or years to decades following their treatment.
- These impairments may include fatigue, pain, neuropathy, lymphedema, or radiation fibrosis syndrome and have the potential to deleteriously impact their function and quality of life.
- Cancer rehabilitation is a comprehensive resource that facilitates maximizing and maintaining cancer survivors' physical, social, psychological, and vocational functioning.
- Application of these services can enhance the ongoing care for cancer survivors.

INTRODUCTION

There are nearly 17 million cancer survivors in the United States, a number expected to exceed 22 million by 2030.[1] At least half of these survivors will experience impairments resulting from their cancer and/or its treatment with potentially significant adverse effects on function and quality of life.[2] The effects of cancer treatment can be long-lasting or even permanent. One study demonstrated that 60% of breast cancer survivors experienced at least 1 or more side effects when assessed at 6 years after diagnosis.[3]

a MedStar Health/Georgetown, National Rehabilitation Hospital, 102 Irving Street Northwest, Washington, DC 20010, USA; b Department of Physical Medicine and Rehabilitation, Rutgers New Jersey Medical School, Kessler Institute for Rehabilitation, 1199 Pleasant Valley Way, West Orange, NJ 07052, USA; c Department of Physical Medicine and Rehabilitation, Rutgers New Jersey Medical School, Select Medical, Kessler Institute for Rehabilitation, 1199 Pleasant Valley Way, West Orange, NJ 07052, USA
* Corresponding author.
E-mail address: mstubblefield@selectmedical.com

Med Clin N Am 104 (2020) 239–250
https://doi.org/10.1016/j.mcna.2019.10.004
0025-7125/20/© 2019 Elsevier Inc. All rights reserved.

This article discusses the principles and practice of comprehensive cancer rehabilitation and its role not only in improving the function and quality of life of cancer survivors, but importantly in providing value to health care as a whole. Specific and commonly seen disorders that benefit from cancer rehabilitation, including fatigue, pain, chemotherapy-induced peripheral neuropathy, lymphedema, and radiation fibrosis syndrome, are discussed.

DEFINITION AND COMPONENTS OF COMPREHENSIVE CANCER REHABILITATION

Cancer rehabilitation is a process that helps cancer survivors obtain and maintain the maximal possible physical, social, psychological, and vocational functioning within the limits created by cancer and its treatments.[4] Models of cancer rehabilitation care delivery and the specific clinicians providing that care vary dramatically across the country.[5] To be truly comprehensive and inclusive of the key skill sets and knowledge to address most functional issues, the rehabilitation team should include physical therapy, occupational therapy, speech language pathology, neuropsychology, cognitive rehabilitation, lymphedema therapy, pelvic floor therapy, and cancer rehabilitation medicine (physiatrist). This minimal core set of cancer rehabilitating specialists is rarely available to the survivors who need them. In fact, many patients struggle to receive treatment from even a single skilled and knowledgeable practitioner regardless of their needs.[6] One study demonstrated that treatment rates for cancer-related functional issues are as low as 1% to 2%.[7]

VALUE OF CANCER REHABILITATION

Historically eradicating cancer and prolonging life (oncology) has been considered more important than restoring function and quality of life (rehabilitation). Improved survival rates and a proliferation of effective treatment options has created an environment in which function and quality of life can be factored into oncologic treatment plans. For many patients, this is not only a consideration, but increasingly a demand. For them, this is the value of cancer rehabilitation.

There is robust evidence for the value of cancer rehabilitation in supporting function and quality of life across a wide range of conditions.[8] When cost is factored in as a major driver of value, then the data are less robust but still favorable for cancer rehabilitation.[9] A more expansive view of the cost-effectiveness value of cancer rehabilitation will be realized if cancer rehabilitation interventions can be proven to decrease emergency room visits and hospitalizations, improve compliance with medications, minimize the oncology team's burden of care, reduce the need for opioids, return patients expeditiously to work, and so forth. Studies demonstrating these value propositions will be key to the adoption and incorporation of comprehensive cancer rehabilitation as standard care in oncology.

BARRIERS TO ACCESS AND HOW TO OVERCOME THEM

Despite the known benefits of cancer rehabilitation, widespread adoption by oncology has yet to be realized. Although there are some exemplary programs, hospitals, and health care systems with quality, multidisciplinary, and comprehensive cancer rehabilitation services, their reach is limited.[6] Lack of knowledge about cancer rehabilitation on the part of patients and referring clinicians further exacerbates referral to and availability of services.[6] Overcoming these barriers will not only take time, but additional research on the value of cancer rehabilitation both clinically and functionally. Patients and clinicians should come to realize that living well beyond cancer is not only possible but should be the expectation for most survivors.

COMMON IMPAIRMENTS IN CANCER SURVIVORS
Relationship Between Cancer and Its Treatments and Functional Impairments

Cancer itself can directly impact body structures and function. These manifestations vary and depend on the location and the extent of disease. Examples may include metastases infiltrating or compressing the lumbosacral plexus resulting in numbness and weakness of the leg[10] or a large lung mass inhibiting pulmonary function and resulting in decreased endurance. Indirectly, cancer can result in paraneoplastic neurologic disorders, such as Lambert-Eaton myasthenic syndrome[11] or paraneoplastic cerebellar degeneration.[12]

Systemic treatments used during cancer treatment include chemotherapy, targeted therapy, immunotherapy, and hormonal therapy. Chemotherapeutic agents, including taxanes, vinca alkaloids, and platinum analogues, may lead to chemotherapy-induced peripheral neuropathy.[13,14] In addition, chemotherapy has been associated with fatigue, cognitive dysfunction, sleep disturbances, and weakness, which can reduce patients' quality of life.[15,16] Targeted therapies interfere with a molecular target to inhibit tumor growth and progression but despite their selectivity, side effects may include interstitial lung disease, cardiotoxicity, hypertension, thromboembolism, skin toxicity, diarrhea, and fatigue.[17] Immunotherapy unleashes the body's immune system and is associated with several neuromuscular adverse events, such as Guillain Barre syndrome, chronic inflammatory demyelinating polyneuropathy, myasthenia gravis, myositis, encephalitis, and brachial plexus neuritis.[18–20] Hormonal therapies can be used in breast and prostate cancer for hormone-sensitive malignancies. Arthralgias are frequently experienced by women on aromatase inhibitors.[21] Androgen deprivation used in prostate cancer can result in fatigue, decline in cognitive function, decreased muscle mass, osteoporosis, and subsequent fractures.[22] Corticosteroids are also commonly used during cancer treatment and may result in myopathy, myalgias, osteoporosis, and osteonecrosis.[23]

Radiation therapy may result in numerous complications. Symptoms vary depending on the tissue involved in the radiation field and may include cognitive dysfunction, myelopathy, and plexopathies.[10] Long-term, radiation fibrosis syndrome can present with myelo-radiculo-plexo-neuro-myopathy, cervical dystonia, neck extensor weakness, trismus, or shoulder pain.[24]

Surgical intervention can alter normal anatomic structures and their function. Neck dissection to treat head and neck cancer can result in spinal accessory nerve palsy and subsequently to shoulder pain.[25] Postmastectomy pain syndrome is a common sequela following surgical intervention for breast cancer.[26] The rehabilitation needs following surgical interventions are unique based on the changes in anatomy, and goals are directed to restoring function.

In addition, another important factor that impacts rehabilitation for patients with cancer is deconditioning. Deconditioning may include generalized weakness, decreased endurance, and exercise intolerance. This can be exacerbated by numerous causes during cancer, including cachexia anemia, fatigue, and generalized immobility leading to muscle atrophy.[27,28]

Cancer and its treatment can result in a multitude of neuromuscular and musculoskeletal disorders that can impair function and impact quality of life. The etiology and manifestations vary broadly, and several examples have been listed previously. Patients may by impacted by multiple complications, and the treatment should be tailored to help maximize their function and improve quality of life while balancing potential risks.

Cancer-Related Fatigue

Cancer-related fatigue is a common symptom that can impact patients from the initial presentation of their cancer, during its treatment, and persist for months to years in survivorship. This can be distressing, with a deleterious impact on function and quality of life. The prevalence of cancer-related fatigue varies in the literature from 25% to 99%.[29] Fatigue is a symptom that historically has been underrecognized and under-treated; this is exemplified by results that 50% of patients did not discuss treatment options for fatigue with their oncologist even though they reported that fatigue more adversely affected their lives than pain.[30] Cancer-related fatigue has been defined by the National Comprehensive Cancer Network as "A distressing, persistent, subjective sense of physical, emotional, and/or cognitive tiredness or exhaustion related to cancer or cancer treatment that is not proportional to recent activity and interferes with usual functioning."[31] Patients may complain of generalized weakness, postexertional malaise, decreased ability to concentrate, emotional reactivity, unrefreshing sleep, insomnia, or hypersomnia.[29,32]

It is imperative to recognize fatigue so that appropriate treatments can be initiated to help decrease this symptom burden and maximize patients' function and quality of life. Comorbidities with potential contributions to fatigue should be treated.[32] Treatment options include exercise, psychosocial interventions, nutritional consultation, sleep therapy, and medications.[29] Exercise is recommended and has been supported by systematic review as a treatment for cancer-related fatigue during and following cancer treatment.[33] Yoga specifically has category 1 evidence as an intervention for cancer-related fatigue.[31] Cognitive behavioral therapy promotes self-care management and has been supported in the literature with category 1 evidence,[29,31,34] and a meta-analysis revealed a small but significant effect for psychological intervention studies[35] for managing fatigue. Psychostimulants also may be used to help manage cancer-related fatigue. There is preliminary evidence for their use; however additional investigation is needed.[36] For patients with more advanced cancer, corticosteroids have been found effective in reducing fatigue,[37] but use is limited because of long-term side effects.

Pain

Pain is a common symptom experienced by cancer survivors, with an estimated prevalence of 66% in patients with advanced disease and 39% following treatment.[38] Pain can be attributed to direct tumor involvement, metastases, or treatment effects, or be unrelated to cancer and its treatment.[39,40] Severe pain can impact function and quality of life.[41] Pain during cancer treatment and survivorship can be attributed to a myriad of etiologic pain generators. Identifying the pain generator(s) is imperative to help guide treatment strategies to decrease pain and maximize function and quality of life. Treatment options to help manage pain can include medications, therapeutic exercise, modalities, and injection procedures.

There are numerous medications to help manage pain. Analgesics may include acetaminophen, nonsteroidal anti-inflammatory drugs (NSAIDs), or opioids. Selecting appropriate medications depends on the etiology of pain. When pain is related to bone metastasis, NSAIDs, bisphosphonates, or radiotherapy may be beneficial.[42] Nerve-stabilizing medications, such as pregabalin and gabapentin are recommended for chemotherapy-induced peripheral neuropathy.[43,44] Additional commonly used medications for neuropathic pain include duloxetine, venlafaxine, amitriptyline, and topical capsaicin.

Physical therapy is commonly used to treat musculoskeletal pain complaints. Therapeutic exercise helps stabilize painful areas and improve myofascial pain.[45] Patients may better tolerate performing isometric contractions that avoid changes in muscle or joint positioning that may produce pain.[46] It can be conducted as outpatient or home-based programs.[47] A systematic review concluded that exercise is beneficial before, during, and after cancer treatment for all cancer types and can improve physical function and assuage impairments.[48] However, safety is a priority, as many patients have comorbidities, such as bone metastases, peripheral neuropathy, or myopathy, and evaluation by a physiatrist can help guide treatment plans to maximize benefit and minimize risk.

Multiple modalities, including heat, cold, and transcutaneous electrical nerve stimulation can be used to help manage pain. Complementary and alternative medicine, such as acupuncture, cupping, music interventions, Chinese herbal medicine, and reflexology may ameliorate cancer pain, but additional studies are needed to confirm their benefits. Bracing, orthotics, assistive devices, and compensatory strategies are also beneficial in mitigating pain.[46]

Depending on the etiology of pain, several types of injections may be considered. Commonly used injectates include corticosteroids, local anesthetics, and botulinum toxins. Dry needling and trigger point injections may be considered for myofascial pain.[45] The efficacy rate of trigger point injections in patients with advanced cancer was found to be 0.59.[49] There are numerous additional injections that may be used to help alleviate pain in cancer survivors, such as botulinum toxin injection for radiation-induced cervical dystonia[50] and intercostobrachial nerve blocks for post-mastectomy pain syndrome[51]; however, expounding on these options is beyond the scope of this article.

On a last note, the management of pain during cancer treatment and survivorship can be complex and may require a multimodal approach individualized to patients based on their etiologic pain generators, comorbidities, prognosis, and preferences.

Chemotherapy-Induced Peripheral Neuropathy

Chemotherapy-induced peripheral neuropathy results from damage and dysfunction of the peripheral nerves. From involvement of motor and sensory nerves, patients may experience numbness, paresthesias, pain, weakness, impaired proprioception, or gait abnormalities. Pain can manifest as dysesthesias or allodynia.[52] When autonomic nerves are affected, patients may experience orthostatic hypotension, constipation, or urinary or sexual dysfunction. These symptoms can result in functional impairments that interfere with performing activities of daily living, decrease quality of life, and may be a dose-limiting toxicity.[52,53]

The incidence of chemotherapy-induced peripheral neuropathy is not fully established, as it varies widely based on the chemotherapeutic agent (6%–100%), dosing, patient comorbidities, and the method of assessment.[52,54] Agents known to be associated with neuropathy are taxanes, vinca alkaloids, platinum compounds, bortezomib, and thalidomide. The manifestation of symptoms may vary based on the agents used and their pathophysiologic mechanisms. Vinca alkaloids and taxanes cause axonal damage by inhibiting microtubules and present with a length-dependent, distal symmetric, motor, and sensory neuropathy.[13,52] Symptoms may present within the first day of treatment,[55] severity increases with dose and duration,[52] and tends to improve over weeks to months when the agents are discontinued.[56] Platinum compounds accumulate within the dorsal root ganglia resulting in DNA damage and present with predominantly sensory symptoms.[14] With high doses, damage also can occur in the anterior horn cell.[57] Another unique feature more common with platinum compounds is "coasting," which describes the phenomenon that symptoms can progress for months following treatment.[58]

A baseline evaluation before neurotoxic chemotherapy has been recommended.[52] It is valuable to identify preexisting conditions that may increase the risk of developing neuropathy. Of particular importance is patients with Charcot-Marie-Tooth, as it has been associated with severe neuropathy following treatment with vincristine.[59,60] History is paramount, and information should be gathered regarding patients' types of symptoms, onset, time course in relation to treatment, distribution, severity, pain assessment, functional assessment, and ability to perform activities of daily living. Laboratory testing can help rule out other potential causes of neuropathy, such as paraneoplastic neurologic disorders, or metabolic or nutritional deficiencies.

Thus far, there is no approved effective treatment for chemotherapy-induced peripheral neuropathy. During chemotherapy, regular monitoring is recommended, as symptoms may progress. Pharmacologic recommendations to address the pain and paresthesias are based on evidence found to be efficacious in painful diabetic neuropathy.[44] Duloxetine[61] and pregabalin[62] have been found to be effective. Additional pharmacologic options include gabapentin, duloxetine, venlafaxine, amitriptyline, valproate, opioids, and capsaicin.[43] Electrical stimulation[63] and acupuncture[64] have been found to decrease pain in small samples of patients with chemotherapy-induced peripheral neuropathy. Symptoms such as numbness and weakness, although not ameliorated by the pharmacologic interventions discussed previously, can be managed with alternative strategies. These include education on fall prevention, therapeutic exercise, lower extremity strengthening, gait and balance training, home modifications, assistive devices, and orthotics.[56,65]

Lymphedema

Cancer and its treatment have the potential to damage lymphatic drainage, resulting in the accumulation of protein-rich lymphatic fluid in the extremities, genitalia, face, neck, or trunk. This secondary lymphedema can present with swelling, pain, sensation of heaviness, and impaired function.[66] Untreated this can progress to lymphostatic elephantitis.[67] Subsequently, alterations in biomechanics can result in secondary neuromuscular and musculoskeletal complications.[68–70]

The reported incidence of lymphedema in the cancer setting varies and has predominantly been reported for breast cancer with rates ranging from 13% to 65%.[71,72] Several cancer treatments can influence the likelihood of developing lymphedema. Chemotherapy as well as radiation therapy involving the lymph nodes increases the risk.[73] Studies have demonstrated that sentinel lymph node biopsy reduces the risk of lymphedema in comparison with axillary lymph node dissection.[74]

The clinical evaluation of lymphedema should include assessment for other causes of peripheral edema, such as hypoalbuminemia, heart failure, chronic venous insufficiency, and severe hypothyroidism (myxedema). It is also imperative to rule out other potentially serious causes of increased limb swelling, such as deep vein thrombosis or tumor recurrence.[75] For this, imagining modalities such as Doppler ultrasound, computed tomography, or MRI with contrast may be indicated.

There are currently several techniques for evaluating lymphedema, including measurement of limb circumference, water displacement, lymphoscintigraphy, perometry, and bioimpedance. Bioimpedance has demonstrated positive results in early assessment with standardized cutoffs and increased sensitivity.[73,76] With earlier identification, patients can benefit from initiation of early treatment strategies and reduce the risk of progression.[77]

Management of lymphedema is aimed at decreasing swelling, improving function, and decreasing secondary complications. Treatment options include complete decongestive therapy, low-level laser therapy, and pharmacologic and surgical intervention.[78] Complete decongestive therapy is commonly recommended[79] and includes manual lymph drainage, compression bandaging, compression garments, exercise, and skin care,[80] with evidence of effectiveness in reducing limb volume[80,81] and improving quality of life.[82] Additional conservative management options include weight management, given the increased risk of lymphedema with obesity,[83,84] and resistance exercise, including weight lifting, which has been demonstrated to reduce lymphedema.[85] Skin hygiene is also crucial to help prevent infections, such as cellulitis, which may require antibiotics and/or antimycotics.[67]

Radiation Fibrosis Syndrome

Radiation fibrosis syndrome encompasses a myriad of symptoms that can occur as a result of tissue fibrosis and sclerosis following radiation therapy. Any tissue type, including the neuromuscular and musculoskeletal systems, can be affected. Symptoms can manifest months, years, or decades after treatment. Sequelae are extremely varied and may include visceral (ie, cardiac, pulmonary, gastrointestinal, integumentary, endocrine, vascular, lymphatic), soft tissue (ie, tendon, ligament, fascia), bone, and neuromuscular dysfunction. Commonly seen neuromuscular disorders include trismus, cervical dystonia, dropped head syndrome, and myelo-radiculo-plexo-neuro-myopathy.[24]

There are many factors that contribute to the risk of developing radiation fibrosis syndrome, including the total dose of radiation, fraction size, treatment field size, tissue types encompassed by the radiation field, and the utilization of additional treatments, such as neurotoxic chemotherapy.[86] There have been several advances in radiation therapy that help minimize the damage to healthy tissue, such as 3-dimensional conformational techniques[87] and intensity-modulated radiotherapy.[87,88]

Radiation fibrosis can impact any portion of the nervous system, including the brain (cerebropathy), spinal cord (myelopathy), nerve roots (radiculopathy), plexus (plexopathy), or peripheral nerves (mononeuropathy). Symptoms may include weakness, sensory change, pain, orthostatic hypotension, or bowel or bladder dysfunction. Muscles also may be affected by radiation and result in a focal myopathy.[89] Patients may present with muscle spasms, muscle weakness, and pain.[24] In addition, radiation fibrosis syndrome may impact multiple structure within the neuromuscular system, referred to as "myelo-radiculo-plexo-neuro-myopathy." This results in a vast array of clinical presentations. Dropped head syndrome or neck extensor weakness exemplifies this.[90] In cervical dystonia, the sternocleidomastoid, trapezius, and scalene muscles are affected, resulting in spasm of the anterior neck, which can progress to contracture and contribute to dysphagia, dysarthria, and difficulty with activities of daily living, such as driving.[24,50,91] Another clinical manifestation is trismus, which is impaired mouth opening, and results from involvement of the trigeminal nerve, masseter, and pterygoid muscles, as well as associated tendons, ligaments, fascia, and skin[24] affecting feeding, oral hygiene, and pulmonary function.[92,93]

Although at this time there is no treatment to reverse the mechanisms underlying radiation fibrosis, treatment is targeted at managing the sequelae and improving and maintaining function and quality of life.[94] Physical therapy is recommended to improve posture, range of motion, strength, endurance, and balance. Patients may benefit from myofascial release or other manual therapies.[94] In addition, treatment is targeted as the specific manifestations. For instance, botulinum toxin injections for cervical dystonia,[50] jaw stretching devices for trismus,[91,95] or cervical collars for dropped head syndrome.[24]

SUMMARY

Providing high-quality, comprehensive, multidisciplinary cancer rehabilitation services is critical to restoring the highest possible level of function and quality of life to cancer

246　Kline-Quiroz et al

survivors. Given the number of possible impairments, teams composed of rehabilitation medicine, physical therapy, occupational therapy, speech language pathology, cognitive rehabilitation, neuropsychology, pelvic floor therapy, and lymphedema therapy, among others, are required to ensure that the patient has access to the suite of services needed. Making the incorporation of cancer rehabilitation the standard of care in oncology will require considerable effort, dedication, and persistence.

DISCLOSURE

None.

REFERENCES

1. Miller KD, Nogueira L, Mariotto AB, et al. Cancer treatment and survivorship statistics, 2019. CA Cancer J Clin 2019;69(5):363–85.
2. Ness KK, Wall MM, Oakes JM, et al. Physical performance limitations and participation restrictions among cancer survivors: a population-based study. Ann Epidemiol 2006;16:197–205.
3. Schmitz KH, Speck RM, Rye SA, et al. Prevalence of breast cancer treatment sequelae over 6 years of follow-up: the pulling through study. Cancer 2012; 118:2217–25.
4. Stubblefield MD, Kendig TD, Khanna A. ReVitalizing cancer survivors—making cancer rehabilitation the standard of care. MD Advis 2019;12:30–3.
5. Cheville AL, Mustian K, Winters-Stone K, et al. Cancer rehabilitation: an overview of current need, delivery models, and levels of care. Phys Med Rehabil Clin N Am 2017;28:1–17.
6. Stubblefield MD. The underutilization of rehabilitation to treat physical impairments in breast cancer survivors. PM R 2017;9:S317–23.
7. Cheville AL, Beck LA, Petersen TL, et al. The detection and treatment of cancer-related functional problems in an outpatient setting. Support Care Cancer 2009; 17:61–7.
8. Stubblefield MD. Cancer rehabilitation—principles and practice. 2nd edition. New York: Demos Medical; 2018.
9. Mewes JC, Steuten LM, Ijzerman MJ, et al. Effectiveness of multidimensional cancer survivor rehabilitation and cost-effectiveness of cancer rehabilitation in general: a systematic review. Oncologist 2012;17:1581–93.
10. Giglio P, Gilbert MR. Neurologic complications of cancer and its treatment. Curr Oncol Rep 2010;12:50–9.
11. Mason W, Graus F, Lang B, et al. Small-cell lung cancer, paraneoplastic cerebellar degeneration and the Lambert-Eaton myasthenic syndrome. Brain 1997; 120:1279–300.
12. Dalmau J, Rosenfeld MR. Paraneoplastic syndromes of the CNS. Lancet Neurol 2008;7:327–40.
13. Lee JJ, Swain SM. Peripheral neuropathy induced by microtubule-stabilizing agents. J Clin Oncol 2006;24:1633–42.
14. Meijer C, de Vries EG, Marmiroli P, et al. Cisplatin-induced DNA-platination in experimental dorsal root ganglia neuronopathy. Neurotoxicology 1999;20:883–7.
15. Love RR, Leventhal H, Easterling DV, et al. Side effects and emotional distress during cancer chemotherapy. Cancer 1989;63:604–12.
16. Kayl AE, Meyers CA. Side-effects of chemotherapy and quality of life in ovarian and breast cancer patients. Curr Opin Obstet Gynecol 2006;18:24–8.

17. Widakowich C, de Castro G Jr, de Azambuja E, et al. Review: side effects of approved molecular targeted therapies in solid cancers. Oncologist 2007;12: 1443–55.

18. Kolb NA, Trevino CR, Waheed W, et al. Neuromuscular complications of immune checkpoint inhibitor therapy. Muscle Nerve 2018;58:10–22.

19. Alhammad RM, Dronca RS, Kottschade LA, et al. Brachial plexus neuritis associated with anti-programmed cell death-1 antibodies: report of 2 cases. Mayo Clin Proc Innov Qual Outcomes 2017;1:192–7.

20. Dalakas MC. Neurological complications of immune checkpoint inhibitors: what happens when you 'take the brakes off' the immune system. Ther Adv Neurol Disord 2018;11. 1756286418799864.

21. Crew KD, Greenlee H, Capodice J, et al. Prevalence of joint symptoms in postmenopausal women taking aromatase inhibitors for early-stage breast cancer. J Clin Oncol 2007;25:3877–83.

22. Kumar RJ, Barqawi A, Crawford ED. Adverse events associated with hormonal therapy for prostate cancer. Rev Urol 2005;7(Suppl 5):S37–43.

23. Frieze DA. Musculoskeletal pain associated with corticosteroid therapy in cancer. Curr Pain Headache Rep 2010;14:256–60.

24. Stubblefield MD. Radiation fibrosis syndrome: neuromuscular and musculoskeletal complications in cancer survivors. PM R 2011;3:1041–54.

25. McNeely ML, Parliament M, Courneya KS, et al. A pilot study of a randomized controlled trial to evaluate the effects of progressive resistance exercise training on shoulder dysfunction caused by spinal accessory neurapraxia/neurectomy in head and neck cancer survivors. Head Neck 2004;26:518–30.

26. Macdonald L, Bruce J, Scott NW, et al. Long-term follow-up of breast cancer survivors with post-mastectomy pain syndrome. Br J Cancer 2005;92:225.

27. Cheville A. Rehabilitation of patients with advanced cancer. Cancer 2001;92: 1039–48.

28. Lakoski SG, Eves ND, Douglas PS, et al. Exercise rehabilitation in patients with cancer. Nat Rev Clin Oncol 2012;9:288–96.

29. Ebede CC, Jang Y, Escalante CP. Cancer-related fatigue in cancer survivorship. Med Clin North Am 2017;101:1085–97.

30. Vogelzang NJ, Breitbart W, Cella D, et al. Patient, caregiver, and oncologist perceptions of cancer-related fatigue: results of a tripart assessment survey. The fatigue coalition. Semin Hematol 1997;34(3 Suppl 2):4–12.

31. Network NCC. Cancer related fatigue (version 2.2019). Available at: https://www.nccn.org/professionals/physician_gls/pdf/fatigue.pdf. Accessed October 23, 2019.

32. Mitchell SA. Cancer-related fatigue: state of the science. PM R 2010;2:364–83.

33. Cramp F, Byron-Daniel J. Exercise for the management of cancer-related fatigue in adults. Cochrane Database Syst Rev 2012;(11):CD006145.

34. van der Lee M, Garssen B. Mindfulness-based cognitive therapy reduces chronic cancer related fatigue: s7-1. Pscyhooncology 2013;22:102–3.

35. Jacobsen PB, Donovan KA, Vadaparampil ST, et al. Systematic review and metaanalysis of psychological and activity-based interventions for cancer-related fatigue. Health Psychol 2007;26:660.

36. Minton O, Richardson A, Sharpe M, et al. Psychostimulants for the management of cancer-related fatigue: a systematic review and meta-analysis. J Pain Symptom Manage 2011;41:761–7.

37. Yennurajalingam S, Frisbee-Hume S, Palmer JL, et al. Reduction of cancer-related fatigue with dexamethasone: a double-blind, randomized, placebo-controlled trial in patients with advanced cancer. J Clin Oncol 2013;31:3076–82.
38. Van Den Beuken-Van MH, Hochstenbach LM, Joosten EA, et al. Update on prevalence of pain in patients with cancer: systematic review and meta-analysis. J Pain Symptom Manag 2016;51:1070–90.e9.
39. Kocoglu H, Pirbudak L, Pence S, et al. Cancer pain, pathophysiology, characteristics and syndromes. Eur J Gynaecol Oncol 2002;23:527–32.
40. Cheville AL. Pain management in cancer rehabilitation. Arch Phys Med Rehabil 2001;82:S84–7.
41. Serlin RC, Mendoza TR, Nakamura Y, et al. When is cancer pain mild, moderate or severe? Grading pain severity by its interference with function. Pain 1995;61:277–84.
42. Ahmad I, Ahmed MM, Ahsraf MF, et al. Pain management in metastatic bone disease: a literature review. Cureus 2018;10:e3286.
43. Bril V, England JD, Franklin GM, et al. Evidence-based guideline: treatment of painful diabetic neuropathy–report of the American Association of Neuromuscular and Electrodiagnostic Medicine, the American Academy of Neurology, and the American Academy of Physical Medicine & Rehabilitation. Muscle Nerve 2011;43:910–7.
44. Stubblefield MD. Cancer rehabilitation. Semin Oncol 2011;38:386–93.
45. Cheville AL, Basford JR. Role of rehabilitation medicine and physical agents in the treatment of cancer-associated pain. J Clin Oncol 2014;32:1691–702.
46. Cheville AL, Smith SR, Basford JR. Rehabilitation medicine approaches to pain management. Hematol Oncol Clin North Am 2018;32:469–82.
47. Su TL, Chen AN, Leong CP, et al. The effect of home-based program and outpatient physical therapy in patients with head and neck cancer: a randomized, controlled trial. Oral Oncol 2017;74:130–4.
48. Stout NL, Baima J, Swisher AK, et al. A systematic review of exercise systematic reviews in the cancer literature (2005-2017). PM R 2017;9:S347–84.
49. Hasuo H, Kanbara K, Abe T, et al. Factors associated with the efficacy of trigger point injection in advanced cancer patients. J Palliat Med 2017;20:1085–90.
50. Stubblefield MD, Levine A, Custodio CM, et al. The role of botulinum toxin type A in the radiation fibrosis syndrome: a preliminary report. Arch Phys Med Rehabil 2008;89:417–21.
51. Wijayasinghe N, Duriaud HM, Kehlet H, et al. Ultrasound guided intercostobrachial nerve blockade in patients with persistent pain after breast cancer surgery: a pilot study. Pain Physician 2016;19:E309–18.
52. Stubblefield MD, Burstein HJ, Burton AW, et al. NCCN task force report: management of neuropathy in cancer. J Natl Compr Canc Netw 2009;7(Suppl 5):S1–26 [quiz: S7–8].
53. Hausheer FH, Schilsky RL, Bain S, et al. Diagnosis, management, and evaluation of chemotherapy-induced peripheral neuropathy. Semin Oncol 2006;33:15–49.
54. Cavaletti G, Alberti P, Frigeni B, et al. Chemotherapy-induced neuropathy. Curr Treat Options Neurol 2011;13:180–90.
55. Holmes FA, Walters RS, Theriault RL, et al. Phase II trial of taxol, an active drug in the treatment of metastatic breast cancer. J Natl Cancer Inst 1991;83:1797–805.
56. Stubblefield MD, McNeely ML, Alfano CM, et al. A prospective surveillance model for physical rehabilitation of women with breast cancer: chemotherapy-induced peripheral neuropathy. Cancer 2012;118:2250–60.
57. Quasthoff S, Hartung HP. Chemotherapy-induced peripheral neuropathy. J Neurol 2002;249:9–17.

58. Siegal T, Haim N. Cisplatin-induced peripheral neuropathy. Frequent off-therapy deterioration, demyelinating syndromes, and muscle cramps. Cancer 1990;66: 1117–23.
59. Hildebrandt G, Holler E, Woenkhaus M, et al. Acute deterioration of Charcot-Marie-Tooth disease IA (CMTIA) following 2 mg of vincristine chemotherapy. Ann Oncol 2000;11:743–7.
60. Igarashi M, Thompson EI, Rivera GK. Vincristine neuropathy in type I and type II Charcot-Marie-Tooth disease (hereditary motor sensory neuropathy). Med Pediatr Oncol 1995;25:113–6.
61. Smith EM, Pang H, Cirrincione C, et al. Effect of duloxetine on pain, function, and quality of life among patients with chemotherapy-induced painful peripheral neuropathy: a randomized clinical trial. JAMA 2013;309:1359–67.
62. Nihei S, Sato J, Kashiwaba M, et al. Efficacy and safety of pregabalin for oxaliplatin- and paclitaxel-induced peripheral neuropathy. Gan To Kagaku Ryoho 2013; 40:1189–93 [in Japanese].
63. Smith TJ, Coyne PJ, Parker GL, et al. Pilot trial of a patient-specific cutaneous electrostimulation device (MC5-A Calmare(R)) for chemotherapy-induced peripheral neuropathy. J Pain Symptom Manage 2010;40:883–91.
64. Wong R, Sagar S. Acupuncture treatment for chemotherapy-induced peripheral neuropathy–a case series. Acupunct Med 2006;24:87–91.
65. Visovsky C, Collins M, Abbott L, et al. Putting evidence into practice: evidence-based interventions for chemotherapy-induced peripheral neuropathy. Clin J Oncol Nurs 2007;11:901–13.
66. Honnor A. Classification, aetiology and nursing management of lymphoedema. Br J Nurs 2008;17:576–86.
67. The diagnosis and treatment of peripheral lymphedema: 2013 consensus document of the International Society of Lymphology. Lymphology 2013;46:1–11.
68. Lin JT, Stubblefield MD. De Quervain's tenosynovitis in patients with lymphedema: a report of 2 cases with management approach. Arch Phys Med Rehabil 2003;84:1554–7.
69. Herrera JE, Stubblefield MD. Rotator cuff tendonitis in lymphedema: a retrospective case series. Arch Phys Med Rehabil 2004;85:1939–42.
70. Stubblefield MD, Custodio CM. Upper-extremity pain disorders in breast cancer. Arch Phys Med Rehabil 2006;87:S96–9 [quiz: S100-1].
71. Kwan ML, Darbinian J, Schmitz KH, et al. Risk factors for lymphedema in a prospective breast cancer survivorship study: the pathways study. Arch Surg 2010; 145:1055–63.
72. Gärtner R, Jensen M-B, Kronborg L, et al. Self-reported arm-lymphedema and functional impairment after breast cancer treatment–a nationwide study of prevalence and associated factors. Breast 2010;19:506–15.
73. Shah C, Arthur D, Riutta J, et al. Breast-cancer related lymphedema: a review of procedure-specific incidence rates, clinical assessment aids, treatment paradigms, and risk reduction. Breast J 2012;18:357–61.
74. Mansel RE, Fallowfield L, Kissin M, et al. Randomized multicenter trial of sentinel node biopsy versus standard axillary treatment in operable breast cancer: the ALMANAC trial. J Natl Cancer Inst 2006;98:599–609.
75. Braddom's physical medicine & rehabilitation. Fifth edition. Philadelphia: Elsevier; 2016.
76. Cornish B, Chapman M, Hirst C, et al. Early diagnosis of lymphedema using multiple frequency bioimpedance. Lymphology 2001;34:2–11.

77. Stout Gergich NL, Pfalzer LA, McGarvey C, et al. Preoperative assessment enables the early diagnosis and successful treatment of lymphedema. Cancer 2008;112:2809–19.

78. Paskett ED, Dean JA, Oliveri JM, et al. Cancer-related lymphedema risk factors, diagnosis, treatment, and impact: a review. J Clin Oncol 2012;30:3726–33.

79. Poage E, Singer M, Armer J, et al. Demystifying lymphedema: development of the lymphedema putting evidence into practice® card. Clin J Oncol Nurs 2008;12: 951–64.

80. Lasinski BB, Thrift KM, Squire D, et al. A systematic review of the evidence for complete decongestive therapy in the treatment of lymphedema from 2004 to 2011. PM R 2012;4:580–601.

81. Karadibak D, Yavuzsen T, Saydam S. Prospective trial of intensive decongestive physiotherapy for upper extremity lymphedema. J Surg Oncol 2008;97:572–7.

82. Kim SJ, Yi CH, Kwon OY. Effect of complex decongestive therapy on edema and the quality of life in breast cancer patients with unilateral lymphedema. Lymphology 2007;40:143–51.

83. Sagen Å, Kåresen R, Risberg MA. Physical activity for the affected limb and arm lymphedema after breast cancer surgery. A prospective, randomized controlled trial with two years follow-up. Acta Oncol 2009;48:1102–10.

84. DiSipio T, Rye S, Newman B, et al. Incidence of unilateral arm lymphoedema after breast cancer: a systematic review and meta-analysis. Lancet Oncol 2013;14: 500–15.

85. Schmitz KH, Ahmed RL, Troxel A, et al. Weight lifting in women with breast-cancer–related lymphedema. N Engl J Med 2009;361:664–73.

86. Cross NE, Glantz MJ. Neurologic complications of radiation therapy. Neurol Clin 2003;21:249–77.

87. Roopashri G, Baig M. Current advances in radiotherapy of head and neck malignancies. J Int Oral Health 2013;5:119.

88. Peng G, Wang T, Yang K-Y, et al. A prospective, randomized study comparing outcomes and toxicities of intensity-modulated radiotherapy vs. conventional two-dimensional radiotherapy for the treatment of nasopharyngeal carcinoma. Radiother Oncol 2012;104:286–93.

89. Portlock CS, Boland P, Hays AP, et al. Nemaline myopathy: a possible late complication of Hodgkin's disease therapy. Hum Pathol 2003;34:816–8.

90. Furby A, Behin A, Lefaucheur J-P, et al. Late-onset cervicoscapular muscle atrophy and weakness after radiotherapy for Hodgkin disease: a case series. J Neurol Neurosurg Psychiatry 2010;81:101–4.

91. Stubblefield MD, Manfield L, Riedel ER. A preliminary report on the efficacy of a dynamic jaw opening device (dynasplint trismus system) as part of the multimodal treatment of trismus in patients with head and neck cancer. Arch Phys Med Rehabil 2010;91:1278–82.

92. Krennmair G, Ulm C, Lenglinger F. Effects of reduced mouth opening capacity (trismus) on pulmonary function. Int J Oral Maxillofac Surg 2000;29:351–4.

93. Scott B, Butterworth C, Lowe D, et al. Factors associated with restricted mouth opening and its relationship to health-related quality of life in patients attending a Maxillofacial Oncology clinic. Oral Oncol 2008;44:430–8.

94. Stubblefield MD. Clinical evaluation and management of radiation fibrosis syndrome. Phys Med Rehabil Clin 2017;28:89–100.

95. Cohen EG, Deschler DG, Walsh K, et al. Early use of a mechanical stretching device to improve mandibular mobility after composite resection: a pilot study. Arch Phys Med Rehabil 2005;86:1416–9.

Cancer Rehabilitation:
Acute and Chronic Issues, Nerve Injury, Radiation Sequelae, Surgical and Chemo-Related, Part 2

Phalgun Nori, MD[a], Cristina Kline-Quiroz, DO[b],
Michael D. Stubblefield, MD[c],*

KEYWORDS

- Postmastectomy pain • Cervical dystonia • Trismus • Brain tumor rehabilitation
- Nontraumatic spinal cord injury

KEY POINTS

- Cancer affects millions of individuals, and approximately half will develop functional impairments.
- Cancers that commonly, either from direct effects or from its treatments, result in functional impairments include breast, head and neck, brain, and spinal cord tumors.
- There is a plethora of potential impairments including pain, spasticity, dystonia, weakness, and neurogenic bowel or bladder.

INTRODUCTION

Physiatrists frequently encounter and manage sequalae from cancer and its treatment. Common cancers with functional impairment treated by physiatrists include breast, head and neck, brain, and spinal cord tumors. The functional complications faced by cancer survivors vary greatly depending on the cancer type and how it was treated. Head and neck cancer survivors, for instance, are commonly treated with surgery, chemotherapy, and radiation therapy. As a result they can develop dysphagia, dysarthria, cervical dystonia, trismus, lymphedema, shoulder dysfunction, and plexopathy among other painful and function-limiting sequelae.[1] Many of these late effects can develop years or even decades following completion of treatment

[a] Department of Physical Medicine and Rehabilitation, Rutgers New Jersey Medical School, Kessler Institute for Rehabilitation, 1199 Pleasant Valley Way, West Orange, NJ 07052, USA; [b] MedStar Health/Georgetown, National Rehabilitation Hospital, 102 Irving Street Northwest, Washington, DC 20010, USA; [c] Department of Physical Medicine and Rehabilitation, Rutgers New Jersey Medical School, Select Medical, Kessler Institute for Rehabilitation, 1199 Pleasant Valley Way, West Orange, NJ 07052, USA
* Corresponding author.
E-mail address: mstubblefield@selectmedical.com

Med Clin N Am 104 (2020) 251–262
https://doi.org/10.1016/j.mcna.2019.10.005   medical.theclinics.com

even if the cancer has been eradicated. Without knowledgeable and skilled cancer rehabilitation clinicians with training in the relevant disciplines, survivors with such diverse impairments are unlikely to realize the maximal possible level of function and quality of life. This article discusses the principles and practice of comprehensive cancer rehabilitation and its role in improving the function and quality of life specific to survivors of breast, head and neck, brain, and spinal cord tumors.

BREAST CANCER

Numerous neuromuscular and musculoskeletal symptoms commonly develop in breast cancer survivors. Approximately 7 out of 8 women with breast cancer experience an upper extremity symptom.[2] The authors highlight shoulder pain, post-mastectomy pain, and aromatase inhibitor arthralgias in this section. Fatigue, chemotherapy-induced peripheral neuropathy, and lymphedema are also commonly seen in breast cancer but are discussed as individual sections. Additional disorders encountered after breast cancer include radiculopathy, plexopathy, mononeuropathies, and epicondylitis.[3]

In the setting of breast cancer treatment there are numerous conditions that contribute to the development of shoulder pain. The prevalence varies but has been reported up to nearly 50%.[4] Patients may guard shoulder movement due to postsurgical pain following breast surgery, axillary dissection, breast reconstruction, or radiation.[5] In addition, there can be nerve damage such as cervical radiculopathy or radiation fibrosis, resulting in weakness in the rotator cuff muscles.[6,7] Axillary web syndrome and lymphedema can also predispose patients to shoulder dysfunction.[8,9] The pectoral muscles can be tightened and shortened altering the shoulder biomechanics, which can lead to rotator cuff tendinopathy and adhesive capsulitis.[6,10] Physical therapy is a mainstay of treatment of both rotator cuff disease and adhesive capsulitis.[3,5] For mild to moderate pain, nonsteroidal antiinflammatories[7] may be helpful. For more severe pain corticosteroid injections[11] may be considered; however, its effect may be small and temporary.

Postmastectomy pain syndrome is defined as "pain that occurs after any breast surgery; is of at least moderate severity; possesses neuropathic qualities; is located in the ipsilateral breast/chest wall, axilla, and/or arm; lasts at least 6 months; occurs at least 50% of the time; and may be exacerbated by movements of the shoulder girdle."[12] More recently it has been referred to as upper quadrant pain.[13] The prevalence historically has varied from 4% to 68%[14,15] and symptoms may persist for up to 12 years in 17%.[14] Although the exact cause is unclear, it is likely related to tissue damage from surgical intervention or radiation with possible direct injury, scar tissue, or neuroma formation[3,7,15] commonly involving the intercostobrachial nerves or branches of the intercostal nerves.[15] Patients may also experience phantom breast sensation or pain.[16] Treatment can include physical therapy for skin desensitization and myofascial release. Mindfulness-based cognitive therapy has been shown to be effective in decreasing late posttreatment pain.[7,17] Pharmacologic options include amitriptyline, venlafaxine, gabapentin, and topical capsaicin.[18,19] Autologous fat grafting and ultrasound-guided intercostobrachial nerve blocks were shown to decrease pain in small studies.[18,20]

Aromatase inhibitors are used for hormone-sensitive breast cancer.[21] Arthralgias may be experienced by nearly 50% of women treated[22] and can be so severe that 13%[23] to 20%[24] interrupted aromatase inhibitor therapy. Aching pain and stiffness may be experienced throughout the body and tenosynovial changes may be present.[25] Preexisting neuromuscular or musculoskeletal disorder may be exacerbated.[3]

Aromatase inhibitors have been associated with carpal tunnel syndrome (median mononeuropathy at the wrist) and potentially additional entrapment syndromes.[26] Currently there are no clinical guidelines for the treatment of aromatase inhibitor–associated arthralgias,[27] but treatment strategies similar to those for fibromyalgia may be used such as aerobic exercise and nerve stabilizing agents.[3] Analgesics including nonsteroidal antiinflammatories, acetaminophen, and opiates have also been used.[28] Vitamin D supplementation,[29] acupuncture,[30] and yoga[31] have been found to improve arthralgia symptoms for women on aromatase inhibitors.

HEAD AND NECK CANCER

Head and neck cancers include several cancer sites such as the oral cavity, larynx, pharynx, tongue, and lip.[32] As a result of head and neck cancers and its treatment patients may develop a variety of neuromuscular and musculoskeletal complications. These may include spinal accessory nerve palsy, shoulder dysfunction, cervical dystonia, dysphagia, dysarthria, and trismus among others.[32]

Shoulder pain is a common symptom occurring in 70% of patients following neck dissection overall and 79% following radial neck dissection.[33] In addition to pain, shoulder forward flexion and abduction range of motion were severely reduced.[33] A unique contribution to shoulder pain in head and neck cancer is spinal accessory nerve palsy that occurs following neck dissection and alters shoulder biomechanics.[32] In addition, radiation treatment can result in damage to the cervical nerve roots, brachial plexus, and peripheral nerves of rotator cuff muscles. Weakness in the rotator cuff muscles also alters shoulder biomechanics and contributes to subacromial impingement, tendinopathy, and adhesive capsulitis.[34] There is evidence from small randomized control trials to support progressive resistance exercise training for patients with head and neck cancer with spinal accessor nerve involvement.[35,36] Otherwise recommendations for treating shoulder pain are those for the general population and can incorporate physical therapy, oral nonsteroidal antiinflammatory or nerve-stabilizing agents, corticosteroid injection, or capsular distension.[32,34]

As previously mentioned, cervical dystonia can be a manifestation of radiation fibrosis syndrome. Injury can involve spinal accessory nerve, cervical nerve roots, or cervical plexus affecting the sternocleidomastoid, scalenes, and trapezius. In addition, damage to these structures can also occur during surgical neck dissection. Patients can present with pain, spasms that can progress to contracture. This can contribute to dysphagia, dysarthria, and difficulty performing activities of daily living.[34] Physical therapy involving range of motion, neuromuscular retraining, and myofascial release is the primary treatment.[32] To address neuropathic pain, nerve-stabilizing agents such as gabapentin, pregabalin, and duloxetine may be trialed.[32] Botulinum toxin injections have demonstrated efficacy in small studies in improving neck motion and decreasing pain.[37,38]

Trismus refers to a limited ability to open the mouth and is defined as less than 35 mm.[39] Trismus can occur due to tumor invasion, surgical intervention, radiation therapy, infection, or osteonecrosis.[40] The prevalence of trismus in head and neck cancers ranges from 28%[41] to 50%[42] with an increased risk when the tumor site involved oropharynx[42] and increased radiation dose.[43] Consequently, patients may have difficulty with feeding, speaking, and oral hygiene, which negatively affect quality of life.[44] Treatment of trismus can include physical therapy and jaw stretching appliances. Jaw stretching devices include stacked tongue depressors, corkscrew devices, the TheraBite Jaw Motion Rehabilitation System, and the Dynasplint Trismus System. TheraBite and Dynasplint have been shown to be effective in improving trismus.[45,46] For associated neuropathic pain, nerve stabilizing medication can be implemented.[32] Pentoxifylline showed a modest improvement in a small trial.[47] Botulinum toxin injection was found to decrease pain but not improve jaw opening.[48] Surgical coronoidectomy was shown to improve trismus in a small sample of patient refractory to physical therapy.[49]

The American Cancer Society has published survivorship care guideline. Regular physical activity with 150 minutes of moderate or 75 minutes of vigorous aerobic exercise and strength training 2 days per week is recommended. Additional recommendations for health promotion include maintaining a healthy weight, dietary counseling, tobacco cessation, and oral care with regular dental follow-up.[32]

BRAIN TUMORS

Brain tumors are diverse group of neoplasms arising from different cells of the central nervous system (CNS) or from systemic cancers that have metastasized to the CNS. Systemic cancers most likely to metastasize to the CNS include lung, breast, colorectal, melanoma, and genitourinary cancers. In approximately 15% of all patients with cancer, the primary tumor metastasizes to the CNS.[50] In adolescents and young adults, primary brain tumors are more common than metastatic tumors.

The incidence rate for primary brain and nervous system tumors in adults is estimated to be 23 per 100,000 persons.[51] An estimated 86,970 new cases of primary malignant and nonmalignant brain and other CNS tumors are expected to be diagnosed in the United States in 2019. This includes an estimated 26,170 primary malignant and 60,800 nonmalignant lesions. Intracranial tumors represent only 2% of all cancers but cause significant disability and confer a disproportionate share of cancer morbidity and mortality. Gliomas account for almost 80% of all primary malignant brain tumors. Glioblastoma is the most frequent histology and accounts for more than 50% of gliomas in all age groups, with an incidence rate among elderly patients of 70 years and older of 17.5 per 100,000 person years.[52]

The treatment of brain tumors has improved considerably with advances in surgical approaches, chemotherapy, radiation therapy, and immunotherapy. These improvements have led to prolonged survival time with the possibility of neurologic consequences.[53] Because brain tumors can be sources of significant functional impairment, patients with brain tumors need rehabilitation services to improve their functional status.

Patient with brain tumor can have various neurologic and functional deficits depending on the tumor size and location as well as the patient's age and comorbidities. Functional deficits associated with brain tumors result from primary tumor effects (destruction of tissue, compression of normal brain, increased intracranial pressure), side effects of treatments (postsurgical tissue loss, steroid myopathy) seizures, and immediate or delayed effects of radiation and chemotherapy. Patients will generally benefit from rehabilitation services following brain tumor surgery to address postsurgical deficits. The postsurgical setting is a pivotal point around which rehabilitation services are organized. Impairments that can arise following tumor resection include hemiparesis, sensorimotor deficits, visual perceptual deficits, cognitive problems, cranial nerve deficits, dysphagia, aphasia, ataxia, and spasticity. In addition to focal neurologic deficits, patients can experience deconditioning from prolonged illness, nutritional compromise, and psychological stress, both for the patient and family. Some patients will require intense inpatient rehabilitation and continued outpatient rehabilitation to maximize their functional potential.

The most common neurologic deficits in patients with brain tumor undergoing acute rehabilitation were described by Mukand[54] and include impaired cognition (80%), weakness (78%), and visual–perceptual impairment (53%), with most patients having multiple impairments. A seminal study found that more than 80% of patients with CNS tumor exhibit rehabilitation needs, the greatest proportion of any tumor type.[55]

Functional recovery is similar in patients with brain tumors as those with acute stroke undergoing acute rehabilitation.[56–58] The literature suggests that the length of stay for inpatient rehabilitation for patients with brain tumor is generally shorter than patients with other brain disorders such as traumatic brain injury and stroke.[59] This may be related to better initial functional status; other possible contributing factors include fewer behavioral sequelae, better social supports, and expedited discharge planning due to prognostic factors. In one study, although functional status improved during rehabilitation, quality-of-life scores did not improve until discharge home.[60] The Functional Independence Measure and disability rating scale are more sensitive than the Karnofsky performance status scale in detecting change in functional status.[60]

Specific rehabilitation interventions depend on the combination of deficits and are generally similar to those used in patients with other causes of brain disorders, such as traumatic brain injury or stroke. Rehabilitation efforts are directed toward goals such as improving bed mobility, transfers, self-care, ambulation, and if necessary, wheelchair training. Strategies are used to promote functional cognition, clear communication, bowel and bladder continence, safe swallowing, adequate nutritional intake, optimal sensory input (including vision and hearing), and restorative sleep. Attention must be paid to prevention of complications related to the primary tumor, and other comorbidities such as pain, neurologic decline, seizure, and depression should be evaluated and treated. The hemiplegic patient will generally benefit from gait training with an assistive device and a brace as an ankle foot orthosis when appropriate. Proper arm positioning, with support of the shoulder to prevent pain in a flaccid or spastic limb should be used. A variety of adaptive equipment is available for individuals who must perform tasks one-handed, such as reachers, sock donners, and elastic shoelaces.

Cognitive dysfunction and attentional deficits are both common and highly disrupting to many individuals with brain tumor. Brain tumors and related treatments can impair cognitive function across many domains and can have an impact on patients' quality of life. Cognitive deficits in patients with brain tumors can be caused by the tumor itself, tumor-related epilepsy, treatment (surgery, radiotherapy, antiepileptics, chemotherapy, or corticosteroids), and psychological distress.[61] Most common cognitive disturbances are deficits in memory (working memory), executive functions (cognitive control and flexibility, cognitive processing speed, visual searching, planning, and foresight), and general attention, above and beyond the effects of age, education, and gender. Cognitive therapy has shown to improve attention and verbal memory and less report of mental fatigue compared with randomized controls.[62] Cognitive rehabilitation therapy is based on the principles of neural plasticity of the brain. It is a type of rehabilitation that offers exercises aimed at improving various domains of cognition such as attention, memory, language, and executive/control of functions. Proper treatment with these therapies can help enhance the social and professional integration of patients.

Individuals with brain tumor have a high incidence of neurologic impairments, resulting in functional deficits for which rehabilitation services are necessary and evidence to date supports as beneficial. The overall care needs are similar to those seen in individuals with other causes of brain disorder, such as stroke or brain trauma, and these include treatment of medical problems such as pain, spasticity, and neurogenic bowel and bladder and the improvement of patients' mobility and activities of daily living. Rehabilitation specialists can help prevent complications, maximize function, and improve the quality of life for patients with brain tumors.

SPINAL CORD TUMORS

Patients with cancer can develop SCI as a direct result of their cancer, its treatment, and other preexisting or acquired conditions. SCI in the cancer setting can result directly from the cancer (epidural, leptomeningeal, or intramedullary tumor) or indirectly from the cancer (paraneoplastic phenomenon) or from treatment of the cancer (radiation, chemotherapy, surgery). Other causes of SCI in patients suffering from cancer include infection (meningitis, epidural abscess, discitis/osteomyelitis), vascular disorder (hemorrhage, infarct), degenerative disorder (spinal stenosis), and metabolic disorders (osteoporotic compression fractures).

Spinal cord tumors can be classified according to their anatomic location. Spinal neoplasms are classified as either extradural or intradural.[63] Intradural and extradural neoplasms are approximately equal in prevalence: 50% to 55% extradural and 40% to 45% intradural.[64] Metastatic disease to spinal cord represents most of the extradural tumors. Symptomatic SCI due to spinal metastasis occurs in up to 5% of all patients with cancer.[65] The vertebral body is the most common site of metastasis within the spine, largely reflecting its volume relative to other spinal structures. Metastatic tumors of the spine are more common than primary spine tumors. Cancers that commonly metastasize to the spine are those of breast, lung, prostate, and kidney.[66] Epidural tumor is the most common cause of SCI in cancer and can arise from the vertebra, enter the spinal canal through the neural foramen, or be deposited in the epidural space. Leptomeningeal metastases occur in 3% to 8% of all patients with cancer and can be associated with significant neurologic dysfunction. The most common tumors that metastasize to the leptomeninges include leukemia, lymphoma, melanoma, breast, and lung cancer (**Boxes 1 and 2**).[67]

Box 1
List of the spinal tumors most commonly found in intradural intramedullary and intradural extramedullary spaces

Intradural (40%–45%)

Intradural intramedullary (15%–33%)—Intramedullary tumors arise within the spinal cord itself

- Ependymoma

- Astrocytoma

- Others include hemangioblastoma, subependymoma, oligodendrogiliomas, ganglionoma, neuroblastoma, teratoma, lipoma, and metastases (lung, breast, melanoma, renal cell, and lymphoma)

- Intradural extramedullary (66%–75%)—Tumors arising within the dura but outside the actual spinal cord

- Nerve sheath tumors (schwannoma and neurofibroma)

- Meningioma

- Myxopapillary ependymoma (conus medullaris and filum terminale)

- Paraganglioma

- Dermoid and epidermoid cysts

- Drop metastases

From Kirshblum S, Lin VW. Spinal cord medicine, 3rd edition. New York: Springer Publishing Company; 2019; with permission.

> **Box 2**
> **List of extradural spinal tumors**
>
> Extradural spinal cord tumors (50%–55%)—Extradural tumors are usually metastatic and most often arise in the vertebral bodies
>
> Metastatic (90%–95%)
>
> - Lung
> - Breast
> - Prostate
> - Lymphoma
> - Primary spinal tumors (5%–10%)
> - Plasma cell tumors (multiple myeloma and plasmacytoma)
> - Hemangioma
>
> *From* Kirshblum S, Lin VW.Spinal cord medicine, 3rd edition. New York: Springer Publishing Company; 2019; with permission.

Initial presentation of spinal tumors can vary widely depending on the location, size, and degree of spread into structures such as dura and nerve roots (**Fig. 1**).[68] Intramedullary tumors are usually associated with signs of myelopathy as well as motor and sensory deficits. Patients with tumors that arise outside of the spinal cord generally present with back pain. Tumors within or extrinsic to the spinal cord can cause symptoms through disruption of normal neural elements and pathways, producing both local and distal effects. Neurologic dysfunction distal to the lesion is due to interruption of ascending and descending spinal cord pathways. The most common sequelae are sensory dysesthesias and muscular weakness. Patients often report progressive difficulty in ambulation. Severe distal sensory loss and sphincter dysfunction also may occur. Although neurologic manifestations may begin unilaterally, they can progress to involve both sides of the spinal cord and thereby produce bilateral symptoms and signs.

Metastatic epidural spinal cord compression is a medical emergency that needs rapid diagnosis and treatment if permanent paralysis is to be prevented: the diagnosis is best made with MRI; and corticosteroids, radiation therapy, and surgery are all established treatments.[69] Pain present only on movement suggests mechanical spinal instability, a finding that requires immediate surgical intervention.[70] Life expectancy following spinal surgery varies with cancer type. A retrospective evaluation of patients with neoplastic SCI admitted for inpatient rehabilitation demonstrated a combined median overall survival time of only 4.1 months from the date of rehabilitation admission to death.[71]

Rehabilitation of cancer survivors with spinal cord injury is a challenging task. The level of injury significantly affects the potential for functional recovery. The degree of functional recovery anticipated in a patient with nonmalignant cause of SCI is generally greater than that anticipated in malignant SCI. This is because patients with cancer tend to develop SCI later in the course of their disease.

The care of patients with acute SCI includes maintenance of ventilation in those with high cervical level of injury. It also includes treatment of pain, autonomic dysregulation, and bowel and bladder dysfunction. Patients are at risk of developing deep vein thrombosis (DVT), pulmonary embolism, pulmonary and urinary tract infections, decubitus pressure ulcers, spasticity, contractures, and osteoporosis. A comprehensive

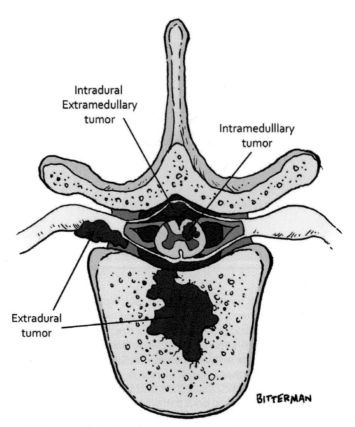

Intradural
Extramedullary
tumor

Intramedulllary
tumor

Extradural
tumor

BITTERMAN

Fig. 1. Anatomic location of spinal cord tumors. (*Courtesy of* Jason Bitterman, MD, Newark, NJ)

treatment plan includes DVT prophylaxis, spirometry and chest physiotherapy, initiation of bowel and bladder program for neurogenic bowel and bladder dysfunction, prevention of decubitus pressure ulcers by turning patient every 2 hours along with use of high-airflow mattresses, use of heel protectors, and daily range of motion exercise.[72,73]

SCI in the cancer setting can present a significant decision-making and management challenge.[74] This challenge is further exacerbated, as cancer-related SCI most often occurs as a late complication when poor overall prognosis and declining medical status can significantly and adversely affect rehabilitation interventions and functional recovery.

SUMMARY

Cancer and its treatment can result in a myriad of functional impairments. The presentations vary depending on the type of cancer and the modalities used in its treatment. Awareness of frequently encountered complications in common cancers can help guide clinicians in identification and treatment. Cancer rehabilitation is a valuable resource to address the functional impairments and improve outcomes of cancer survivors. Efforts should be made to incorporate comprehensive cancer rehabilitation for all cancer survivors who have ongoing sequalae from the disease and treatment.

DISCLOSURE

The authors has nothing to disclose.

REFERENCES

1. Stubblefield MD. Clinical evaluation and management of radiation fibrosis syndrome. Phys Med RehabilClin N Am 2017;28:89–100.
2. McCredie MR, Dite GS, Porter L, et al. Prevalence of self-reported arm morbidity following treatment for breast cancer in the Australian Breast Cancer Family Study. Breast 2001;10:515–22.
3. Stubblefield MD, Keole N. Upper body pain and functional disorders in patients with breast cancer. PMR 2014;6:170–83.
4. Tengrup I, Tennvall-Nittby L, Christiansson I, et al. Arm morbidity after breast-conserving therapy for breast cancer. ActaOncol 2000;39:393–7.
5. McNeely ML, Binkley JM, Pusic AL, et al. A prospective model of care for breast cancer rehabilitation: postoperative and postreconstructive issues. Cancer 2012; 118:2226–36.
6. Ebaugh D, Spinelli B, Schmitz KH. Shoulder impairments and their association with symptomatic rotator cuff disease in breast cancer survivors. Med Hypotheses 2011;77:481–7.
7. Stubblefield MD, Custodio CM. Upper-extremity pain disorders in breast cancer. Arch Phys Med Rehabil 2006;87:S96–9 [quiz:S100–1].
8. Herrera JE, Stubblefield MD. Rotator cuff tendonitis in lymphedema: a retrospective case series. Arch Phys Med Rehabil 2004;85:1939–42.
9. Torres Lacomba M, Mayoral Del Moral O, CoperiasZazo JL, et al. Axillary web syndrome after axillary dissection in breast cancer: a prospective study. BreastCancer Res Treat 2009;117:625–30.
10. Cheville AL, Tchou J. Barriers to rehabilitation following surgery for primary breast cancer. J SurgOncol 2007;95:409–18.
11. Buchbinder R, Green S, Youd JM. Corticosteroid injections for shoulder pain. CochraneDatabaseSyst Rev 2003;(1):CD004016.
12. Waltho D, Rockwell G. Post–breast surgery pain syndrome: establishing a consensus for the definition of post-mastectomy pain syndrome to provide a standardized clinical and research approach—a review of the literature and discussion. Can J Surg 2016;59:342.
13. Cheville AL, McLaughlin SA, Haddad TC, et al. Integrated rehabilitation for breast cancer survivors. Am J Phys Med Rehabil 2019;98:154–64.
14. Macdonald L, Bruce J, Scott NW, et al. Long-term follow-up of breast cancer survivors with post-mastectomy pain syndrome. Br J Cancer 2005;92:225.
15. Jung BF, Ahrendt GM, Oaklander AL, et al. Neuropathic pain following breast cancer surgery: proposed classification and research update. Pain 2003;104:1–13.
16. Dijkstra PU, Rietman JS, Geertzen JH. Phantom breast sensations and phantom breast pain: a 2-year prospective study and a methodological analysis of literature. Eur J Pain 2007;11:99–108.
17. Johannsen M, O'Connor M, O'Toole MS, et al. Efficacy of mindfulness-based cognitive therapy on late post-treatment pain in women treated for primary breast cancer: a randomized controlled trial. J ClinOncol 2016;34:3390–9.
18. Larsson IM, AhmSørensen J, Bille C. The post-mastectomy pain syndrome—a systematic review of the treatment modalities. Breast J 2017;23:338–43.

19. Amr YM, Yousef AA. Evaluation of efficacy of the perioperative administration of venlafaxine or gabapentin on acute and chronic postmastectomy pain. Clin J Pain 2010;26:381–5.

20. Wijayasinghe N, Duriaud HM, Kehlet H, et al. Ultrasound guided intercostobrachial nerve blockade in patients with persistent pain after breast cancer surgery: a pilot study. Pain Physician 2016;19:E309–18.

21. NetworkNCC. Breast cancer (version 3.2019). Available at: https://www.nccn.org/professionals/physician_gls/pdf/breast.pdf. Accessed October 23, 2019.

22. Crew KD, Greenlee H, Capodice J, et al. Prevalence of joint symptoms in postmenopausal women taking aromatase inhibitors for early-stage breast cancer. J ClinOncol 2007;25:3877–83.

23. Henry NL, Giles JT, Ang D, et al. Prospective characterization of musculoskeletal symptoms in early stage breast cancer patients treated with aromatase inhibitors. BreastCancer Res Treat 2008;111:365–72.

24. Fontaine C, Meulemans A, Huizing M, et al. Tolerance of adjuvant letrozole outside of clinical trials. Breast 2008;17:376–81.

25. Morales L, Pans S, Paridaens R, et al. Debilitating musculoskeletal pain and stiffness with letrozole and exemestane: associated tenosynovial changes on magnetic resonance imaging. BreastCancer Res Treat 2007;104:87–91.

26. Nishihori T, Choi J, DiGiovanna MP, et al. Carpal tunnel syndrome associated with the use of aromatase inhibitors in breast cancer. ClinBreastCancer 2008;8:362–5.

27. Winters-Stone KM, Schwartz AL, Hayes SC, et al. A prospective model of care for breast cancer rehabilitation: bone health and arthralgias. Cancer 2012;118:2288–99.

28. Gaillard S, Stearns V. Aromatase inhibitor-associated bone and musculoskeletal effects: new evidence defining etiology and strategies for management. BreastCancer Res 2011;13:205.

29. Rastelli AL, Taylor ME, Gao F, et al. Vitamin D and aromatase inhibitor-induced musculoskeletal symptoms (AIMSS): a phase II, double-blind, placebo-controlled, randomized trial. BreastCancer Res Treat 2011;129:107–16.

30. Crew KD, Capodice JL, Greenlee H, et al. Randomized, blinded, sham-controlled trial of acupuncture for the management of aromatase inhibitor-associated joint symptoms in women with early-stage breast cancer. J ClinOncol 2010;28:1154–60.

31. Galantino ML, Desai K, Greene L, et al. Impact of yoga on functional outcomes in breast cancer survivors with aromatase inhibitor-associated arthralgias. IntegrCancerTher 2012;11:313–20.

32. Cohen EE, LaMonte SJ, Erb NL, et al. American Cancer Society head and neck cancer survivorship care guideline. CA Cancer J Clin 2016;66:203–39.

33. Dijkstra PU, van Wilgen PC, Buijs RP, et al. Incidence of shoulder pain after neck dissection: a clinical explorative study for risk factors. Head Neck 2001;23:947–53.

34. Stubblefield MD. Radiation fibrosis syndrome: neuromuscular and musculoskeletal complications in cancer survivors. PMR 2011;3:1041–54.

35. McNeely ML, Parliament M, Courneya KS, et al. A pilot study of a randomized controlled trial to evaluate the effects of progressive resistance exercise training on shoulder dysfunction caused by spinal accessory neurapraxia/neurectomy in head and neck cancer survivors. Head Neck 2004;26:518–30.

36. McNeely ML, Parliament MB, Seikaly H, et al. Effect of exercise on upper extremity pain and dysfunction in head and neck cancer survivors: a randomized controlled trial. Cancer 2008;113:214–22.

37. Bach C-A, Wagner I, Lachiver X, et al. Botulinum toxin in the treatment of post-radiosurgical neck contracture in head and neck cancer: a novel approach. Eur Ann OtorhinolaryngolHead Neck Dis 2012;129:6–10.
38. Stubblefield MD, Levine A, Custodio CM, et al. The role of botulinum toxin type A in the radiation fibrosis syndrome: a preliminary report. Arch Phys Med Rehabil 2008;89:417–21.
39. Dijkstra P, Huisman P, Roodenburg J. Criteria for trismus in head and neck oncology. Int J Oral MaxillofacSurg 2006;35:337–42.
40. Dhanrajani P, Jonaidel O. Trismus: aetiology, differential diagnosis and treatment. Dent Update 2002;29:88–94.
41. Pauli N, Johnson J, Finizia C, et al. The incidence of trismus and long-term impact on health-related quality of life in patients with head and neck cancer. ActaOncol 2013;52:1137–45.
42. Weber C, Dommerich S, Pau HW, et al. Limited mouth opening after primary therapy of head and neck cancer. OralMaxillofacSurg 2010;14:169–73.
43. Teguh DN, Levendag PC, Voet P, et al. Trismus in patients with oropharyngeal cancer: relationship with dose in structures of mastication apparatus. Head Neck 2008;30:622–30.
44. Kent ML, Brennan MT, Noll JL, et al. Radiation-induced trismus in head and neck cancer patients. Support Care Cancer 2008;16:305–9.
45. Shulman DH, Shipman B, Willis FB. Treating trismus with dynamic splinting: a cohort, case series. AdvTher 2008;25:9–16.
46. Cohen EG, Deschler DG, Walsh K, et al. Early use of a mechanical stretching device to improve mandibular mobility after composite resection: a pilot study. Arch Phys Med Rehabil 2005;86:1416–9.
47. Chua DT, Lo C, Yuen J, et al. A pilot study of pentoxifylline in the treatment of radiation-induced trismus. Am J ClinOncol 2001;24:366–9.
48. Dana MH, Cohen M, Morbize J, et al. Botulinum toxin for radiation-induced facial pain and trismus. OtolaryngolHead Neck Surg 2008;138:459–63.
49. Bhrany AD, Izzard M, Wood AJ, et al. Coronoidectomy for the treatment of trismus in head and neck cancer patients. Laryngoscope 2007;117:1952–6.
50. Schouten LJ, Rutten J, Huveneers HA, et al. Incidence of brain metastases in a cohort of patients with carcinoma of the breast, colon, kidney, and lung and melanoma. Cancer 2002;94:2698–705.
51. Ostrom QT, Gittleman H, Truitt G, et al. CBTRUS statistical report: primary brain and other central nervous system tumors diagnosed in the United States in 2011–2015. Neurooncology 2018;20:iv1–86.
52. Minniti G, Lombardi G, Paolini S. Glioblastoma in elderly patients: current management and future perspectives. Cancers (Basel) 2019;11:336.
53. Huang ME, Sliwa JA. Inpatient rehabilitation of patients with cancer: efficacy and treatment considerations. PMR 2011;3:746–57.
54. Mukand JA, Blackinton DD, Crincoli MG, et al. Incidence of neurologic deficits and rehabilitation of patients with brain tumors. Am J Phys Med Rehabil 2001;80:346–50.
55. Lehmann J, DeLisa J, Warren C, et al. Cancer rehabilitation: assessment of need, development, and evaluation of a model of care. Arch Phys Med Rehabil 1978;59:410–9.
56. Geler-Kulcu D, Gulsen G, Buyukbaba E, et al. Functional recovery of patients with brain tumor or acute stroke after rehabilitation: a comparative study. J ClinNeurosci 2009;16:74–8.

57. Huang ME, Cifu DX, Keyser-Marcus L. Functional outcome after brain tumor and acute stroke: a comparative analysis. Arch Phys Med Rehabil 1998;79:1386–90.
58. O'Dell MW, Barr K, Spanier D, et al. Functional outcome of inpatient rehabilitation in persons with brain tumors. Arch Phys Med Rehabil 1998;79:1530–4.
59. Greenberg E, Treger I, Ring H. Rehabilitation outcomes in patients with brain tumors and acute stroke: comparative study of inpatient rehabilitation. Am J Phys Med Rehabil 2006;85:568–73.
60. Huang ME, Wartella JE, Kreutzer JS. Functional outcomes and quality of life in patients with brain tumors: a preliminary report. Arch Phys Med Rehabil 2001;82: 1540–6.
61. Gehrke AK, Baisley MC, Sonck AL, et al. Neurocognitive deficits following primary brain tumor treatment: systematic review of a decade of comparative studies. J Neurooncol 2013;115:135–42.
62. Gehring K, Sitskoorn MM, Gundy CM, et al. Cognitive rehabilitation in patients with gliomas: a randomized, controlled trial. J ClinOncol 2009;27:3712–22.
63. Chamberlain MC. Salvage chemotherapy for recurrent spinal cord ependymona. Cancer 2002;95:997–1002.
64. Arnautovic K, Arnautovic A. Extramedullaryintradural spinal tumors: a review of modern diagnostic and treatment options and a report of a series. Bosn J Basic Med Sci 2009;9:S40.
65. Parsch D, Mikut R, Abel R. Postacute management of patients with spinal cord injury due to metastatic tumour disease: survival and efficacy of rehabilitation. Spinal Cord 2003;41:205.
66. Ecker RD, Endo T, Wetjen NM, et al. Diagnosis and treatment of vertebral column metastases. MayoClinProc 2005;80(9):1177–86. Elsevier.
67. DeAngelis LM, Boutros D. Leptomeningeal metastasis. Cancer Invest 2005;23: 145–54.
68. Kirshblum S, Lin VW. Spinal cord medicine. 3rd edition. New York: Springer Publishing Company; 2019.
69. Cole JS, Patchell RA. Metastatic epidural spinal cord compression. LancetNeurol 2008;7:459–66.
70. Harel R, Angelov L. Spine metastases: current treatments and future directions. Eur J Cancer 2010;46:2696–707.
71. Guo Y, Young B, Palmer JL, et al. Prognostic factors for survival in metastatic spinal cord compression: a retrospective study in a rehabilitation setting. Am J Phys Med Rehabil 2003;82:665–8.
72. Wuermser L-A, Ho CH, Chiodo AE, et al. Spinal cord injury medicine. 2. Acute care management of traumatic and nontraumatic injury. Arch Phys Med Rehabil 2007;88:S55–61.
73. Kelly BM, Yoder BM, Tang CT, et al. Venous thromboembolic events in the rehabilitation setting. PM R 2010;2:647–63.
74. Stubblefield MD, Bilsky MH. Barriers to rehabilitation of the neurosurgical spine cancer patient. J SurgOncol 2007;95:419–26.

Management of the Patient with Chronic Spinal Cord Injury

Binnan Ong, DO, MSBE[a,b], James R. Wilson, DO[a,b], M. Kristi Henzel, MD, PhD[a,b],*

KEYWORDS

- Spinal cord injuries • Neurogenic bowel • Neurogenic bladder
- Autonomic dysreflexia • Spasticity • Primary health care

KEY POINTS

- Changes in one body system of the patient can have broad implications on a spinal cord–injured patient's function and risk for complications.
- Multidisciplinary management is usually required to achieve optimal health outcomes.
- Physiatrists add special value in evaluating and coordinating complex needs for patients with spinal cord injuries or disorders.

INTRODUCTION

Individuals with spinal cord injuries or disorders (SCI/D) require multidisciplinary care management to achieve optimal health outcomes.Because SCI/D is relatively rare in the general population, primary care providers (PCPs) may not have extensive experience managing people with these disorders. SCI/D impairs the body's autonomic and biomechanical performance by interrupting communications between the brain, organ systems, muscles, and bone. This carries important implications on the patient's ability to perform basic activities of daily living (ADLs) and their reserve capacity to withstand illnesses, procedures, and effects of aging.[1] For PCPs, it is important to recognize that disease presentations, differential diagnoses (**Table 1**), and management may differ from neurologically intact individuals.[2]

PHYSIOLOGY

In SCI/D, location and severity of the lesion determine a person's deficits. Structures innervated from above the cord lesion generally remain functionally intact, whereas structures innervated at or below the lesion are potentially affected. The severity of

[a] Spinal Cord Injuries and Disorders Center, Louis Stokes Cleveland VA Medical Center, 10701 East Boulevard, 128(W), Cleveland, OH 44106, USA; [b] Department of Physical Medicine and Rehabilitation, Case Western Reserve University, MetroHealth System, Old Brooklyn Campus, 4229 Pearl Road, Cleveland, OH 44109, USA
* Corresponding author. Spinal Cord Injuries and Disorders Center, Louis Stokes Cleveland VA Medical Center, 10701 East Boulevard, 128(W), Cleveland, OH 44106.
E-mail address: Mary.henzel@va.gov

Med Clin N Am 104 (2020) 263–278
https://doi.org/10.1016/j.mcna.2019.10.006
0025-7125/20/Published by Elsevier Inc.
medical.theclinics.com

Table 1
Differential diagnoses for common signs and symptoms after spinal cord injury

Sign/Symptom	Causes
Fever[a]	Infection Poikilothermia/hot environment Deep venous thrombosis Heterotopic ossification Pathologic fracture Drug fever Neurogenic "quad" fever Intrathecal baclofen withdrawal[b]
Altered mental status	Medication side effect Infection Renal failure/insufficiency Dehydration Posterior reversible encephalopathy syndrome Seizures Intrathecal baclofen overdose/withdrawal[b]
Fatigue	Nonspecific, may be only symptom of illness Medication side effect Infection Heart failure/coronary artery disease Respiratory failure/insufficiency Depression Hypothyroidism
Daytime drowsiness	Medication side effect Sleep apnea Respiratory dysfunction Depression
Dyspnea	Pneumonia Mucous plugging Abdominal distention/ileus/constipation Pulmonary embolism Respiratory insufficiency Heart failure/coronary artery disease
Diarrhea	Change in bowel program Infection Encopresis (diarrhea around fecal impaction) Medication side effect
Rectal bleeding	Hemorrhoids Bowel care–related trauma Colorectal cancer
Hematuria	Urinary tract infection (UTI) Urinary stones Traumatic catheterization Bladder cancer
Headache	Autonomic dysreflexia Cerebral hemorrhage Typical headache causes

(continued on next page)

Table 1 (continued)	
Sign/Symptom	Causes
Increased spasticity	UTI
	Skin breakdown
	Fecal impaction
	Seating or positioning problems
	Any painful stimulus
	Syrinx
	Intrathecal baclofen withdrawal[b]
Shoulder pain	Rotator cuff tear
	Tendinopathy
	Degenerative joint disease
	Cervical radiculopathy
	Pulmonary embolism
	Syrinx
	Referred visceral pain
	Referred pain from myofascial trigger points
Unilateral limb swelling	Fracture
	Deep venous thrombosis
	Heterotopic ossification
	Cellulitis
	Hematoma
	Cancer-related lymphedema
New weakness or numbness	UTI (triggers increased spasticity)
	Syrinx
	Peripheral neuropathy
	Radiculopathy
	Intrathecal baclofen overdose[b]

[a] Note: basal body temperature may be lower after SCI. "Low-grade" temperature elevations may be significant.
[b] If intrathecal baclofen pump present.
   Adapted from Sabharwal S. Medical complications and consequences of SCI: Overview. In: Essentials of Spinal Cord Medicine. New York: Demos Medical Publishing, LLC; 2014; with permission.

the lesion determines the degree of disruption to the organ's function. Autonomic innervation is particularly important, as it mediates control of thermoregulation, the heart, blood vessels, respiratory tract, gastrointestinal (GI) tract, and urinary bladder among others. Some autonomic innervations are discussed as the authors cover common medical problems facing individuals with SCI/D and introduce the broader context and interdisciplinary management required for optimal care.

Neurogenic Respiratory Dysfunction

The most common cause of death after SCI/D is pneumonia and respiratory diseases.[3] Respiratory dysfunction occurs due to inspiratory muscle weakness, impaired cough due to expiratory muscle weakness (**Table 2**), and decreased surfactant production.[4] It is compounded by complications of SCI/D, for example, abdominal distention from constipation resisting diaphragmatic movement. Injuries above T6 cause impaired sympathetic outflow, and unopposed vagal tone, via the vagus nerve, results in increased bronchial secretions and bronchoconstriction.

Higher injury levels result in greater respiratory compromise with tetraplegics carrying the greatest risk of pneumonia morbidity, mucous plugging, respiratory failure, and sleep-disordered breathing. Late-onset ventilatory failure may also occur due to

Table 2
Respiratory muscle innervation and function

Respiratory Muscle	Innervation	Respiratory Function
Diaphragm	C3–C5 via phrenic nerve	Inhalation
Intercostals	T1–T11 via intercostal nerves	Inhalation, exhalation, cough
Abdominals	T6–T12	Exhalation, cough
Trapezius and sternocleidomastoid	Cranial nerve XI, C2–C4	Inhalation
Scalenes	C4–C8	Inhalation

age-related changes in alveoli and vital capacity; restrictive deficits from reduced chest wall and lung compliance, obesity, and kyphoscoliosis; and neurologic decline.[1]

Annual evaluation and optimization of respiratory health for at-risk individuals includes radiographs, pulmonary function tests, polysomnography (if snoring or somnolence are noted), and offering influenza and pneumococcal vaccinations. Aggressive and routine pulmonary toileting is important especially when individuals develop respiratory infections (**Table 3**).[5] The most underutilized modality is mechanical insufflation-exsufflation, aka "Cough Assist," which mimics cough physiology: providing a positive pressure breath via mouthpiece or tracheostomy adapter followed by sudden negative pressure to clear respiratory secretions.[6] Unlike tracheal suction, this does not cause or worsen mucosal irritation.

DIAGNOSING AND TREATING RESPIRATORY INFECTIONS

Compared with neurologically intact individuals, those with SCI/D can pose a diagnostic challenge because respiratory muscle weakness masks typical symptoms of dyspnea, tachypnea, and cough. Hypotension, hypoxemia, tachypnea, and altered

Table 3
Strategies for prevention and treatment of atelectasis and pneumonia

Problem	Assistive Devices	Medications
Atelectasis	Mechanical Insufflation/ exsufflation Incentive spirometer Positive end-expiratory pressure devices Noninvasive or invasive ventilation	Bronchodilators
Mucous secretions	Mechanical insufflation/ exsufflation Chest physiotherapy Chest wall oscillation vest Flutter valve	Nebulized normal saline Nebulized hypertonic (3%) saline Nebulized acetylcysteine Bronchodilators
Insufficient ventilation	Noninvasive ventilation (CPAP/BiPAP/AVAPS) Invasive home ventilation Diaphragmatic pacing systems	Theophylline
Decreased surfactant	Mechanical insufflation for hyperinflation	Long-acting beta agonists Short-acting beta agonists Theophylline

mental status are commonly the only presenting symptoms. Because of high morbidity, hospitalization is recommended particularly in high tetraplegia. Aggressive pulmonary toileting (see **Table 2**), antibiotics, and close respiratory function monitoring should be provided.[7]

Cardiovascular Autonomic Dysfunction

In chronic SCI/D, sympathetic control of the heart and peripheral blood vessels can be altered, whereas parasympathetic control via the vagus nerve is preserved.[8] The resulting vasoconstrictive and chronotropic dysregulation results in:

- Low basal blood pressures,
- Orthostatic hypotension, and
- Autonomic dysreflexia

Low basal blood pressure occurs due to loss of tonic sympathetic peripheral vasoconstriction. In tetraplegia, asymptomatic systolic blood pressures around 90 mm Hg are common. It is important, therefore, to identify the individual's baseline blood pressure to determine if a low reading is truly pathologic and to guide treatment endpoints with fluids or pressors.

Orthostatic hypotension is common early after tetraplegia but tends to improve over time. The inability to mobilize vascular volumes by sympathetically vasoconstricting blood vessels causes an ineffective baroreceptor reflex due to blood pooling in the splanchnic vasculature and dependent extremities. Reflexive parasympathetic inhibition compensates by increasing heart rate; however, this is often inadequate to increase cardiac output. Treatments include progressive postural challenge, fluid resuscitation, abdominal binders, compression stockings, midodrine, ephedrine, and fludrocortisone.

Autonomic dysreflexia (AD) is a *medical emergency* unique to spinal cord injuries above the T6 level. It manifests as a sudden increase in blood pressure 20 to 40 mm Hg higher than the adult patient's baseline in response to noxious stimuli below the level of injury. A "normal" blood pressure of 120/80 may represent AD in tetraplegics whose baseline systolic pressures are commonly 90 mm Hg. Severe AD can increase systolic pressures to greater than 200 mm Hg and cause myocardial infarction, cerebral hemorrhage, seizures, and death. Symptoms can include headache, sweating, and flushing above the level of injury, piloerection, blurry vision, nasal congestion, and bradycardia, but many are asymptomatic. Overdistention of the bladder or bowel is the most common trigger, although surgical intervention, restrictive clothing, ingrown toenails, fractures, sexual intercourse, menstruation, and labor are other potential causes. AD is important to recognize even at benign absolute blood pressures, as it may be the only cue to prompt a workup in someone with impaired sensation. The treatment is to remove or palliate the painful stimulus (eg, treatment algorithm in **Fig. 1**). Blood pressure rapidly returns to baseline once the noxious stimulus is resolved or palliated; however, short-acting antihypertensives are sometimes necessary.

Cardiovascular Disease

The fourth most common cause of death after SCI/D is hypertensive and ischemic heart disease.[3] Unsurprisingly, people with SCI/D have multiple risk factors for cardiovascular disease (CVD), including low high-density lipoprotein, inactivity, obesity related to lower metabolic rates, and glucose intolerance.[9]

In cervical and high thoracic lesions, blunted cardiac pain afferents from T1 to T5 can result in acute coronary syndrome without chest pain. Only nonspecific

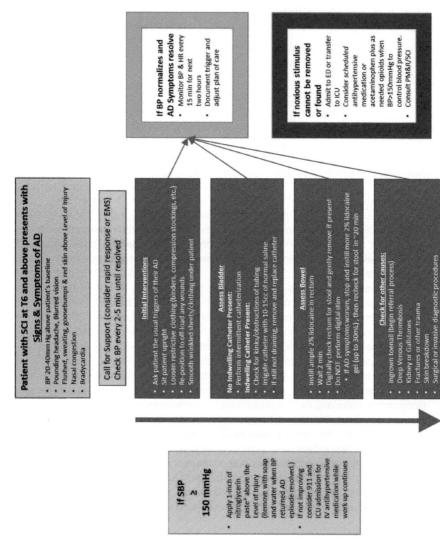

Fig. 1. Example of autonomic dysreflexia protocol.[a] Use alternative if phosphodiesterase-5 inhibitors taken in past 24 hours.

symptoms such as dyspnea, AD, nausea, spasticity, or syncope may be present, resulting in delayed diagnosis. Likewise, peripheral vascular disease may only present as a nonhealing limb wound, because claudication is typically absent. Risk factor evaluation including nicotine use and lipid management is recommended every 3 years after SCI. Because of inability to achieve sufficient cardiac stress with arm ergometry, chemical stress tests are usually required if there is suspicion for inducible ischemia.

Thermoregulation

SCI/D impairs thermoregulation due to altered hypothalamic control, inability to sweat or shiver, and poor vasomotor tone. In high tetraplegia, poikilothermia—the inability to maintain a constant core temperature independent of ambient temperature—can be seen. Fever and hypothermia must consequently be carefully interpreted[10]:

- Basal body temperatures in tetraplegia may be 1 to 2°F lower than normal, so low-grade or borderline fevers may be significant.
- Excessive blankets or high ambient room temperatures can mimic fever.
- Heat stroke and hypothermia are greater possibilities.

Metabolic and Endocrine Dysfunction

Metabolic and endocrine function is altered after SCI/D and should be considered in medical decision-making[11]:

- *Sarcopenic obesity* results from lower basal metabolic rates, osteoporosis, and the inability to exercise paralyzed muscles. This reduces lean body mass and increases adiposity making standard body mass index cutoffs inaccurate. Metabolic syndrome is more prevalent after SCI/D and, in severe cases, may require bariatric surgery to achieve weight loss.
- *Hypercalcemia and hypercalciuria* occur for the first 6 to 18 months after SCI due to immobility-related bone resorption.
- *Hyponatremia* may occur in chronic tetraplegia. Its cause is unclear, but fluid restriction may be needed.
- *Testosterone deficiency* is more common in young men with SCI/D than the general population. Cause is likely central at hypothalamus and pituitary.
- *Osteoporosis* occurs with increased fragility fractures and low-trauma injuries. Bone density imaging should be performed. Further study is needed to optimally prevent and treat SCI/D-related bone loss. Secondary causes of osteoporosis such as vitamin D deficiency, which is more common after SCI, hyperparathyroidism, hyperthyroidism, and hypogonadism, should be screened for and treated.

Neurogenic Bowel Dysfunction

Lower GI symptoms occur in most of the patients with SCI, resulting in increased morbidity and decreased quality of life. Social isolation, malnutrition from poor appetite, skin breakdown from fecal incontinence, and AD are potential complications of a poorly regulated bowel.[12]

Essential GI functions including peristalsis and mucosal secretions are regulated directly by the enteric nervous system and indirectly by sympathetic and parasympathetic control.[12,13] Sympathetic output from T5 to L2 levels decreases peristalsis and secretions. Parasympathetic tone promotes digestion but notably has split innervation. Vagal tone modulates the proximal GI system from esophagus up to the transverse colon, whereas sacral S2 to S4 levels control the distal colon and rectum. Although upper GI dysfunction can occur after SCI/D, the greatest clinical impairment is in the distal colon where autonomic tone is purely spinally derived. Somatic control of the anal sphincter—mediated by the pudendal nerve (S2–S4)—may be impaired at any spinal level, resulting in altered tone and voluntary control.

BOWEL MANAGEMENT PROGRAM

Management of neurogenic constipation requires a program that provides for scheduled bowel movements at least 3 times per week, with intervening continence.[12,14] Fluid intake, diet, medications, physical function, anorectal tone, anal reflexes, independence with bowel care, and caregiver support should all be taken into consideration. Medication management is driven by the bowel phenotype (**Box 1**). Evaluate for common constipating agents, that is, opioids and anticholinergics, and consider alternatives whenever possible.

Promotility agents such as senna are used when the patient is having infrequent or insufficient bowel movements, but higher doses decrease time for colonic water resorption and may excessively soften stool.

Softeners such as docusate modify stool consistency but may improve stool motility slightly secondarily due to greater ease of peristalsis.

Evacuants trigger rectocolonic reflex contractions or use mechanical means to remove stool in those unable to initiate a bowel movement:

- Digital rectal stimulation: using a gloved and lubricated finger to stretch the internal anal sphincter and trigger reflexive distal colonic peristalsis.[13]
- Magic bullet suppositories (water-soluble bisacodyl): preferred over other formulas.[12]
- Docusate mini-enema: more effective than suppositories in comparative studies.[15]

Box 1
Neurogenic bowel phenotypes

Upper Motor Neuron "Spastic" Bowels
  Most commonly seen in SCI/D lesions above conus medullaris.
  Uncoordinated peristalsis decreases bowel motility.
  Spastic anal sphincter provides some continence.
  Intact sacral reflexes allow digital rectal stimulation and/or suppositories to trigger stool evacuation.
  Stool should be kept soft but formed for ease of passage.

Lower Motor Neuron "Flaccid" Bowels
  Seen in spinal shock, cauda equina syndrome, or other peripheral nerve pathology.
  Poor anorectal tone, absent sacral reflexes.
  Decreased bowel motility in the distal colon.
  Low anorectal tone causes incontinence at low abdominal pressures, for example, during Valsalva or position changes.
  Lack of reflexive distal colonic contractions makes digital stimulation and suppositories ineffective.
  Stool is manually disimpacted or flushed out with large-volume enemas.
  Stool should be kept formed and firm for ease of manual evacuation.

Data from Stiens SA, Bergman SB, Goetz LL. Neurogenic bowel dysfunction after spinal cord injury: Clinical evaluation and rehabilitative management. Arch Phys Med Rehabil 1997;78(3 Suppl):S86-102.

- Manual evacuation/disimpaction: manually removing stool piece-by-piece for flaccid bowels.
- Large-volume enemas loosen and flush stool out if manual evacuation is incomplete.

Diverting ileostomy or colostomy can be considered if a patient has the following[12,14,16]:

- Inability to achieve continence despite optimizing the bowel program.
- Excessive bowel program duration.
- Impaired wound healing due to fecal contamination.
- Insufficient function or caregivers to perform bowel program.
- Recurrent AD due to chronic constipation.

ACUTE ABDOMEN

Because of impaired abdominal sensation, high clinical suspicion for acute abdominal pathologies is also needed. Conditions including appendicitis, bowel obstruction/ileus, peptic ulcers, cholelithiasis, and pancreatitis may present with only nonspecific symptoms such as fever, nausea, or AD, leading to delayed diagnosis.[12]

Neurogenic Voiding Dysfunction

After SCI/D, several common patterns of voiding dysfunction may occur (**Table 4**).[17]
Decreased bladder capacity and elasticity is common with chronic neurogenic dysfunction, leading to urinary urgency, leakage, dangerous filling/voiding pressures, and AD even at "normal" or low urinary volumes. A urodynamics study is needed to assess bladder pressures, outlet obstruction, and voiding function.[17,18]

MEDICATIONS

Bladder medications are prescribed based on the cause of the patient's symptoms.[17,19] Detrusor overactivity may be treated with anticholinergics, β_3-agonist mirabegron, or intravesicular botulinum toxin injections. Detrusor-sphincter dyssynergia and prostatic outlet obstruction may be treated with α_1 antagonists or 5α-reductase inhibitors. PCPs should be cognizant that constipation, orthostasis, and sexual dysfunction are common at baseline in the SCI population and may be worsened by side effects from these medications.

Table 4 Neurogenic bladder dysfunction	
Detrusor overactivity (DO)	• Reflexive and uninhibited bladder contraction during filling. • Detrusor and urinary sphincter contraction balance determines continence
Detrusor sphincter dyssynergia (DSD)	• External urethral sphincter co-contraction with detrusor • Elevated detrusor pressures may threaten upper urinary tracts
Flaccid/atonic bladder	• Seen during spinal shock, sacral spinal injuries, or peripheral nerve lesions • Compliant bladder stores large volumes before exceeding urethral sphincter pressure • Detrusor cannot contract to empty completely, if at all

VOIDING TECHNIQUES

Voiding methods are selected based on neuro-urologic and hand function, ability to manage clothing, and caregiver support.[19] Clean intermittent catheterization is ideal for those with adequate hand function, bladder capacity, and discipline to adhere to a catheterization schedule. Indwelling catheters are convenient for those unable to intermittently catheterize but are associated with more frequent infections, urinary stones, and decreased bladder capacity. External catheters may be used by volitional or reflexive voiders who lack adequate hand function for clothing management but requires verification of safe voiding pressures and amenable body habitus.[17]

BACTERIURIA AND URINARY TRACT INFECTIONS

No gold standard exists for diagnosing urinary tract infections (UTIs) in neurogenic bladders because asymptomatic bacteriuria (ASB) develops quickly.[17,20,21] ASB is practically inevitable in individuals using invasive catheterization. Markers of UTI for the nonneurogenic population are highly prevalent in asymptomatic individuals using intermittent and indwelling catheters, including nitrites, leukocyte esterase, and pyuria. Therefore, urinalyses and culture should not be screened in asymptomatic patients. The *absence* of pyuria, however, is a strong negative predictor and should prompt evaluation of alternative diagnoses in symptomatic patients. Studies show that patients are only roughly 50% accurate in predicting if they have a UTI and commonly use poor predictors such as cloudiness or malodorous urine. The Infectious Diseases Society of America (IDSA) lists neurogenic bladder UTI symptoms as follows in **Box 2**.

Symptomatic UTI in the setting of neurogenic bladder remains a clinical diagnosis that is ruled-in by the presence of significant bacteriuria, at least one sign or symptom of UTI, and no other obvious cause. The IDSA defines a colony count of greater than or equal to 10^3 CFU/mL from a fresh catheter specimen or midstream voided urine specimen as significant if there are UTI symptoms.[20] When testing for UTI, change any indwelling catheter before obtaining a urine sample and start empirical antibiotics based on local resistance patterns. Tailor antibiotics based on culture sensitivities

---

Box 2
Urinary tract infection symptoms in neurogenic bladder

- Fever
- Fatigue/malaise/lethargy with no identifiable cause
- Altered mental status
- Dysuria (if sensation intact)
- Hematuria
- Abdominal/suprapubic/costovertebral discomfort (if sensation intact)
- New or worsening urinary leakage
- New or worsening spasticity
- Autonomic dysreflexia

Data from Hooton TM, Bradley SF, Cardenas DD, et al. Diagnosis, Prevention, and Treatment of Catheter-Associated Urinary Tract Infection in Adults: 2009 International Clinical Practice Guidelines from the Infectious Diseases Society of America. Clin Infect Dis 2010;50(5):625-663.

once available. Antibiotic duration is 5 to 14 days with the longer duration recommended for those with more severe presenting symptoms.

Patients having more than 2 UTIs a year should be evaluated for urinary stone disease, poor catheterization technique, incomplete emptying, and bladder overdistension. The routine use of prophylactic antibiotics for recurrent UTI is not recommended. Cranberry juice and methenamine are commonly used prophylactic agents with minimal side effects, which lack strong evidence.[20]

The IDSA recommends that ASB *should* be treated with targeted antibiotics for 1 to 2 doses just before urologic surgeries.[21]

UPPER URINARY TRACT SURVEILLANCE

Hydronephrosis and renal failure may complicate inadequate urinary drainage and should prompt urologic referral. In severe cases, patients may require urinary diversions or bladder augmentation to preserve renal function. Patients with SCI/D should have their upper urinary tracts evaluated regularly; however, optimal screening intervals and methods (kidney and bladder ultrasound, computed tomography [CT], renal nuclear scan, etc.) are not well established.[17,19] Creatinine clearance is an insensitive measure of renal function in SCI/D due to muscle atrophy, and 24-hour clearance may be needed.[17]

Impaired Skin Integrity

Skin breakdown causes significant morbidity and mortality in people with SCI/D. There is a 50% to 80% lifetime risk for pressure injuries (PrIs), which can be attributed to numerous predisposing risk factors including the following[22,23]:

- Decreased muscle tone and mass
- Decreased vascular response to mechanical load
- Poor sensation of early tissue compromise
- Limited ability to reposition self
- Compromised skin integrity due to stool and urine incontinence
- Comorbid conditions (diabetes, tobacco, dyslipidemia, malnutrition, etc.)
- Reliance on well-fitted and well-maintained support surfaces to mitigate risk

Similar to the neurologically intact population, wound care begins with the assessment and optimization of nutritional status, micronutrient deficiency, tobacco cessation, and medical comorbidity management.[23] Osteomyelitis should be suspected in any chronic nonhealing wound. Wound bed management including evaluation for osteomyelitis is similar to neurologically intact patients but falls outside the scope of this article. A few unique SCI/D considerations are mentioned in the following section.

SUPPORT SURFACES

Because of inability to reposition themselves, people with high paraplegia and tetraplegia are reliant on well-maintained support surfaces. In bed, advanced support mattresses and heel suspension boots should be used.[24,25] The ideal wheelchair seating configuration and cushion selection should be determined by a wheelchair seating specialist with SCI/D experience.[22,23] Wheelchair cushions breakdown over time and should be replaced when they exceed their functional lifespan. Even temporary changes in weight (eg, pregnancy), range of motion, and function (eg, pain or deconditioning from illness) may require seating system adjustments to optimize skin health and mobility.

PRESSURE RELIEF STRATEGIES

People who cannot reposition themselves regularly should be turned in bed by caregivers every 2 to 4 hours on an appropriate support surface.[23,24,26] Lying on firm surfaces including gurneys, examination tables, or a malfunctioning air mattress can cause or worsen PrIs in susceptible individuals. Side-lying positions should be limited to a 30° incline to minimize pressure on bony prominences.[24] When supine, head of bed elevation should be less than 30° or be accompanied by elevation of the patient's legs to decrease shearing across the sacrum. Wheelchair users should be educated in off-loading techniques such as forward leans in manual chairs or tilting in power chairs to redistribute pressure.[26] Pressure relief intervals vary based on the patient's risk of PrI. Generic recommendations are 1 minute every 15 to 30 minutes while seated; however, full tissue reperfusion can take up to 3 minutes.[27] Development or worsening of a PrI should warrant reevaluation of the support surfaces, increase in pressure relief frequency, or temporary full-time bedrest.

Chronic Pain

Chronic pain is common after SCI/D, affecting ∼80% of patients.[28] Classification schema often center around pain quality, location, and severity. Pain quality narrows the classification into neuropathic or nociceptive. Above-level pain is typically nociceptive due to traumatic injuries or overuse disorders. At-level neuropathic pain follows dermatomal patterns due to neuronal injury at the injured spinal segment. Below-level pain is classically neuropathic type pain and difficult to treat; however visceral, radicular, and nociceptive pain types also occur.

NEUROPATHIC PAIN

Mechanisms underlying neuropathic pain are incompletely understood but may result from central or peripheral nervous system injury. Treatments (**Table 5**) focus on preventing triggers, promoting central reinterpretation, downregulating receptors, or suppressing peripheral nerve activity.

Table 5
Neuropathic pain management

Priority	Options
First-line, minimal side effects	• Desensitization therapies • Orthotics (eg, compression gloves) • Cognitive behavioral therapy • Gate theory–mediated modalities (eg, transcutaneous electrical nerve stimulation, massage)
Second-line oral medications	• Gabapentinoids • Antidepressants (SNRI and tricyclics)
Third-line oral medications	• Other antiepileptic medications • Tramadol may be helpful for short-acting pain relief due to its SNRI effects
Adjuvant medication options	• Topicals (eg, anesthetics or capsaicin) • Acetaminophen • Nonsteroidal antiinflammatory drugs (NSAIDs) • Antispasticity medications

Abbreviation: SNRI, serotonin and norepinephrine reuptake inhibitor.

Opioids have limited efficacy and should be avoided due to risk of opioid-induced hyperalgesia. Side-effect profiles, drug interactions, and insurance coverage frequently dictate medication selection, but recent recommendations suggest pregabalin, the only medication with a Food and Drug Administration indication for SCI-related neuropathic pain, is the appropriate first choice when available.[29] Interventional procedures and surgeries are reserved for recalcitrant cases and should be performed by providers experienced in the postoperative needs and anticipated outcomes of individuals with SCI.

SHOULDER PAIN/OVERUSE SYNDROMES

Individuals with SCI/D place heavy loads on their upper limbs during transfers, wheelchair propulsion, and ADLs, which occur at a mechanical disadvantage due to wheelchair-level positioning, impaired trunk stability, and potential arm weakness. Shoulder pain, rotator cuff injury, and carpal tunnel syndrome are very common in the SCI population. Prevention should be emphasized since the incidence of rotator cuff injury increases with duration of wheelchair use.[30] Shoulder pain should trigger rapid referral to an SCI/D provider, therapist, and seating specialist, as limited use of even one arm can render a paraplegic dependent for mobility and transfers. Bracing, transition to powered mobility, and behavioral modifications are possible treatment options.[31]

Spasticity

Spasticity is defined as "disordered sensory-motor control, resulting from an upper motor neuron lesion [in the brain or spinal cord], presenting as intermittent or sustained involuntary activation of muscles." Its clinical manifestations include clonus, spasms, spastic cocontraction, and muscle weakness.[32] Loss of central inhibition results in exaggerated stretch reflexes and muscle hyperexcitability such that involuntary muscle spasms occur with small movements. Spasticity typically presents 3 to 6 months post-injury as spinal shock resolves and the UMN syndrome manifests. Spasticity eventually reaches a chronic plateau, and deviations from this baseline should serve as "red flags" to prompt further workup or referral to an SCI provider. Triggers such as UTI or PrI are common but any noxious stimuli may contribute. Spasticity must be differentiated from non-neurologic causes of "tightness" and "spasm" such as contracture, muscle guarding, or misinterpreted neuropathic or radicular pain as the treatments differ.

Potentially positive effects of spasticity include decreased muscle atrophy, increased metabolism, and improved tissue blood flow and ADL function. Treatments are guided by patient-directed functional goals and the avoidance of secondary complications. Stretching and range of motion may be adequate for some people. Treatment often starts with oral baclofen or tizanidine due to superior side effect profiles. Adjuvant medications such as neuropathic pain medications, dopaminergics, opioids, and others may be beneficial in select cases. Medication side effects are common including cognitive complaints and respiratory impairment. Selection of medications and invasive procedures such as chemodenervation with botulinum toxins, intrathecal baclofen pumps, orthopedic contracture release, and neurosurgical interventions such as nerve transfers or dorsal rhizotomies should be guided by the physiatrist.

Musculoskeletal Complications

Because weakness and spasticity often lead to limb immobilization in particular positions, joint contractures are common after SCI/D. Contractures should be prevented by proper positioning, bracing, and routine stretching, as they can result in abnormal pressure distribution leading to skin breakdown or difficulty performing ADLs such as perineal hygiene. Spasticity should be treated if present but long-standing contractures or severe deformities often require surgical correction. SCI specialists may trial diagnostic nerve blocks, chemodenervation procedures, and/or serial casting in certain cases.

Lifetime incidence of long bone fractures is as high as 70% and most commonly occurs around the knee joint. These are often provoked by simple ADLs, twisting, or stretching and may present as vague symptoms similar to deep vein thrombosis (DVT) or cellulitis. Increased spasticity or AD may be seen.[11] Treatment may be conservative (splinting or casting) or aggressive (open fixation) depending on functional status and medical comorbidities. When patients are nonambulatory and osteoporotic/osteopenic, nonoperative treatment may seem enticing. However, prolonged immobilization and orthopedic bracing has profound impact on function, wheelchair positioning, pressure injury risk, AD, caregiver burden, and community participation. Referral to an SCI specialist and SCI-experienced orthopedist is important to avoid long-standing consequences and optimize function.

Heterotopic ossification (HO) occurs when bone forms in periarticular soft tissues. It occurs anywhere below the level of injury, usually 1 to 6 months after SCI/D, and is most commonly found at the anteromedial hip. Symptoms mimic occult fracture or DVT. The clinical impact ranges from negligible to joint ankylosis. A triple phase bone scan is the test of choice. Early diagnosis and prompt referral are vital to ensure the best chance for effective medical treatment. Long-term sequalae can include loss of function, skin breakdown, or neurovascular compromise. Surgical correction can result in reduced range of motion of hip joint and alter seating.[11]

Acute Neurologic Changes

New neurologic changes are concerning and should prompt workup and intervention. Neurologic decline can manifest as ascending motor or sensory deficits, spasticity changes, scoliosis, increased pain, joint deformities, and any unexpected change in function. Unique neurologic sequalae include syringomyelia, arachnoiditis, and tethered cord syndrome. SCI specialists can assist in differentiating these from common peripheral nerve entrapments, musculoskeletal changes, and overuse injuries previously described. Workup includes exclusion of other causes (eg, radiculopathy, infection, tumor) and often MRI or CT myelogram. Suspected cases should be referred to an experienced neurosurgeon for further evaluation.[33]

SUMMARY

Management of SCI/D is unique due to its inherently multidisciplinary and comprehensive nature. SCI/D-related impairments cross multiple organ systems with potentially devastating effects on physical, psychological, and social well-being. Physiatrists, and specifically board-certified SCI Medicine subspecialists, are trained to anticipate, recognize, and manage the deficits that arise throughout the course of a spinal cord–injured person's life. Seemingly isolated problems such a joint pain or incontinence often require a multifaceted approach incorporating therapist evaluations, education, medication management, durable medical equipment modification, and social work coordination to optimize patient outcomes. Because of the unique needs of this population, we recommend that all individuals with SCI/D be established with a physiatrist to coordinate their care across the various medical specialties and ensure treatment decisions consider the entire biopsychosocial context in which they occur.

DISCLOSURE

The authors are salaried clinical employees of the Veterans Health Administration.

REFERENCES

1. Frontera JE, Mollett P. Aging with spinal cord injury: an update. Phys Med RehabilClin N Am 2017;28(4):821–8.
2. Sabharwal S. Medical complications and consequences of SCI: overview. In: Essentials of spinal cord medicine. New York: Demos Medical; 2014. p. 229–31.
3. National Spinal Cord Injury Statistical Center. Complete public version of the 2018 annual statistical report for the spinal cord injury model systems. Available at: https://www.nscisc.uab.edu/public/2018%20Annual%20Report%20-%20Complete%20Public%20Version.pdf. Accessed July 9, 2019.
4. Zimmer MB, Nantwi K, Goshgarian HG. Effect of spinal cord injury on the respiratory system: basic research and current clinical treatment options. J SpinalCord Med 2007;30:319–30.
5. Zakrasek EC, Nielson JL, Kosarchuk JJ, et al. Pulmonary outcomes following specialized respiratory management for acute cervical spinal cord injury: a retrospective analysis. Spinal Cord 2017;55(6):559–65.
6. Consortium for Spinal Cord Medicine. Respiratory management following spinal cord injury: a clinical practice guideline for health-care professionals. Washington, DC: Publisher Paralyzed Veterans of America; 2005.
7. Darouiche RO. Infections in persons with spinal cord injury. In: Kirshblum S, Lin V, editors. Spinal cord medicine. 3rd edition. New York: Demos Medical; 2019. p. 269–77.
8. Sabharwal S. Cardiovascular dysfunction in spinal cord disorders. In: Kirshblum S, Lin V, editors. Spinal cord medicine. 3rd edition. New York: Demos Medical; 2019. p. 212–29.
9. Consortium for Spinal Cord Medicine. Identification and management of cardiometabolic risk after spinal cord injury. Washington, DC: Publisher Paralyzed Veterans of America; 2018.
10. Sabharwal S. Impaired thermoregulation. In: Essentials of spinal cord medicine. New York: Demos Medical; 2014. p. 280–2.
11. Bauman WA, Nash MS. Endocrinology and metabolism of persons with spinal cord injury. In: Kirshblum S, Lin V, editors. Spinal cord medicine. 3rd edition. New York: Demos Medical; 2019. p. 278–317.
12. Vernese LF, Chen D, Anschel A. Gastrointestinal disorders in spinal cord injury. In: Kirshblum S, Lin V, editors. Spinal cord medicine. 3rd edition. New York: Demos Medical; 2019. p. 387–410.
13. Stiens SA, Bergman SB, Goetz LL. Neurogenic bowel dysfunction after spinal cord injury: clinical evaluation and rehabilitative management. Arch Phys Med Rehabil 1997;78(3 Suppl):S86–102.
14. Clinical practice guidelines: neurogenic bowel management in adults with spinal cord injury. Spinal Cord Medicine Consortium. J SpinalCord Med 1998;21(3):248–93.
15. Amir I, Sharma R, Bauman W, et al. Bowel care for individuals with spinal cord injury: comparison of four approaches. J SpinalCord Med 1998;21(1):21–4.
16. Boucher M, Dukes S, Bryan S, et al. Early colostomy formation can improve independence following spinal cord injury and increase acceptability of bowel management. Top SpinalCordInjRehabil 2019;25(1):23–30.

17. Linsenmeyer TA. Urologic management and renal disease in spinal cord injury. In: Kirshblum S, Lin V, editors. Spinal cord medicine. 3rd edition. New York: Demos Medical; 2019. p. 332–86.

18. Weld KJ, Graney MJ, Dmochowski RR. Differences in bladder compliance with time and associations of bladder management with compliance in spinal cord injured patients. J Urol 2000;163(4):1228–33.

19. Consortium for Spinal Cord Medicine. Bladder management for adults with spinal cord injury: a clinical practice guideline for health-care providers. J SpinalCord Med 2006;29(5):527–73.

20. Hooton TM, Bradley SF, Cardenas DD, et al. Diagnosis, prevention, and treatment of catheter-associated urinary tract infection in Adults: 2009 international clinical practice guidelines from the Infectious Diseases Society of America. Clin Infect Dis 2010;50(5):625–63.

21. Nicolle LE, Gupta K, Bradley SF, et al. Clinical practice guideline for the management of asymptomatic bacteriuria: 2019 Update by the infectious diseases Society of America. Clin Infect Dis 2019;68(10):e83–110.

22. Henzel MK, Bogie K. Medical management of pressure injuries in patients with spinal cord disorders. In: Kirshblum S, Lin V, editors. Spinal cord medicine. 3rd edition. New York: Demos Medical; 2019. p. 516–43.

23. Consortium for Spinal Cord Injury Medicine. Pressure ulcer prevention and treatment following spinal cord injury: a clinical practice guideline for health-care professionals. 2nd edition. Washington, DC: Publisher Paralyzed Veterans of America; 2014.

24. National Pressure Ulcer Advisory Panel, European Pressure Ulcer Advisory Panel and Pan Pacific Pressure Injury Alliance. Prevention and treatment of pressure ulcers: clinical practice guideline. Osborne Park (Western Australia): Cambridge Media; 2014.

25. Mcinnes E, Jammali-Blasi A, Bell-Syer SE, et al. Support surfaces for pressure ulcer prevention. Cochrane Database Syst Rev 2015;(9):CD001735.

26. Groah SL, Schladen M, Pineda CG, et al. Prevention of pressure ulcers among people with spinal cord injury: a systematic review. PMR 2014;7(6):613–36.

27. Coggrave MJ, Rose LS. A specialist seating assessment clinic: changing pressure relief practice. Spinal Cord 2003;41(12):692–5.

28. Bryce TN. Pain management in persons with spinal cord injury. In: Kirshblum S, Lin V, editors. Spinal cord medicine. 3rd edition. New York: Demos Medical; 2019. p. 438–56.

29. Guy SD, Mehta S, Casalino A, et al. The CanPain SCI clinical practice guidelines for rehabilitation management of neuropathic pain after spinal cord: recommendations for treatment. Spinal Cord 2016;54(Suppl1):S14–23.

30. Akbar M, Balean G, Brunner M, et al. Prevalence of rotator cuff tear in paraplegic patients compared with controls. JBoneJointSurg Am 2010;92(1):23–30.

31. Paralyzed Veterans of America Consortium for Spinal Cord Medicine. Preservation of upper limb function following spinal cord injury: a clinical practice guideline for health-care professionals. J SpinalCord Med 2005;28(5):434–70.

32. Walker HW, Hon A, Hess MJ. Spasticity management. In: Kirshblum S, Lin V, editors. Spinal cord medicine. 3rd edition. New York: Demos Medical; 2019. p. 472–86.

33. Sarmey N, Lee BS, Benzel EC. Spine complications in patients with spinal cord injury. In: Kirshblum S, Lin V, editors. Spinal cord medicine. 3rd edition. New York: Demos Medical; 2019. p. 559–66.

Neck Pain and Lower Back Pain

Adrian Popescu, MD[a],*, Haewon Lee, MD[b]

KEYWORDS

- Neck pain • Natural history • Treatment • Diagnosis • Physical examination
- Lower back pain • Spine interventions • Red flags

KEY POINTS

- History and physical examination along with risk factors should dictate further needs for imaging for patients with neck or lower back pain.
- A cross-imaging study like MRI should be considered in patients with history of cancer, red flag signs, progressive neurologic deficits, determining the acuity of a fracture, and for presurgical or preprocedural evaluation.
- For patients with acute neck pain who receive appropriate treatment, most cases will resolve over a period of weeks to months.
- Preferential direction of movement in patients with radicular or axial lower back pain symptoms can guide patient's ergonomics and a physical therapy program.
- Seeing a physiatrist spine specialist within 1 week of symptoms onset can increase patient satisfaction, decrease use of care and reduce rates of fusion spine surgeries for patients with lower back pain.

NECK PAIN
Epidemiology

Neck pain is the fourth leading cause of disability.[1] Adult population (ages 15–74 years) shows a point prevalence ranging from 5.9%[2] to 38.7%.[3] The 1-year prevalence of neck pain in the elderly population ranges between 8.8%[4] and 11.6%.[5,6] Females report neck pain more frequently than males.[7,8]

The causes of neck pain vary broadly, with leading causes being inadequate ergonomics at work, sitting and maintaining neck posture in a nonphysiologic position for long periods of time. Duration of symptoms may classify the neck pain as acute at less than 6 weeks, subacute at 3 months or less, or chronic at more than 6 months. There is an association between a shorter duration of neck pain and better prognosis for long-term outcomes.[9,10]

[a] Department of Physical Medicine and Rehabilitation, Hospital of the University of Pennsylvania, Perelman School of Medicine, 1800 Lombard Street, Philadelphia, PA 19146, USA;
[b] Physical Medicine & Rehabilitation, Department of Orthopedic Surgery, University of California San Diego, 200 West Arbor Drive, #8894, San Diego, CA 92103, USA
* Corresponding author.
E-mail address: popescad@uphs.upenn.edu

Med Clin N Am 104 (2020) 279–292
https://doi.org/10.1016/j.mcna.2019.11.003   medical.theclinics.com
0025-7125/20/Published by Elsevier Inc.

Acute neck pain largely resolves within 2 months from the initial pain episode, but a significant proportion of patients continue to have neck pain recurrence or some discomfort at 1 year. The best predictor of future neck pain is presence of an episode of neck pain in the past.[11,12]

Factors associated with neck pain chronicity include psychopathology, low work satisfaction, sedentary lifestyle, headaches, female sex, secondary gain, and poor work physical environment and ergonomics.[13]

Classification

Nontraumatic neck pain can be classified according to the suspected pain generator. It can have a mechanical component (cervical intervertebral disc, cervical zygapophyseal joints, facet joints, ligaments, and atlantoaxial joints), or a neuropathic component (radiculopathy secondary to compression or irritation of the spinal nerve secondary to a disc herniation, foraminal stenosis, or central spinal stenosis), or a combination of both. The controversial entity of myofascial pain syndrome is a condition that probably encompasses neck pain not explained by imaging findings, in a chronic fashion. Neck pain with a neurologic deficit can be cause by disc herniation with nerve root compression, severe foraminal stenosis or disc-osteophyte complex that leads to nerve root compression, or central stenosis leading to cord compression and myelopathy. Ossification of the posterior longitudinal ligament is a unique condition that can cause cord compression and myelopathy. Myelopathy is a clinical diagnosis. It often refers to weakness, balance, and fine motor deficits secondary to spinal cord compression. The differential diagnosis for neck pain is broad and should be used in a diagnostic algorithm: coronary artery disease, infection (osteomyelitis, discitis, retropharyngeal abscess, meningitis, fracture of the dens), malignancy (multiple myeloma, metastatic disease), rheumatologic conditions (polymyalgia rheumatica, calcium pyrophosphate deposition disease at the atlanto-axial joint, fibromyalgia), vascular etiologies (vertebral or carotid dissection), and thoracic outlet syndrome for neck pain associated with arm symptoms. Albeit rare, neck pain conditions that are associated with red flags (myelopathy, osteomyelitis, discitis, bowel or bladder incontinence, suspected malignancy) need to be addressed in a timely fashion and usually require advance imaging (MRI or computed tomography [CT]) along with specific laboratory work (erythrocyte sedimentation rate, C-reactive protein, complete blood count, etc).

History and Physical Examination

The history and physical examination plays a key role in ruling out some of the more serious causes for neck pain that require physician intervention. Differentiating among various painful conditions involving the neck is less critical, especially if the symptoms resolve with time and conservative treatment. Any significant trauma to the head or neck resulting in severe pain should be assessed using the Canadian C-spine rules and NEXUS criteria.[14,15]

Observation of neck and head position and range of motion are an integral part of the physical examination. The clinician should also ask the patient to point to where the pain is perceived, name aggravating and alleviating factors, describe the character of the pain (dull, lancinating, sharp, electric, radiating vs nonradiating), as well as the extent of which the pain is interfering with sleep, driving, working, and activities of daily living. Any antalgic positions of the neck along with restrictions in active and passive range of motions should be noted. Cervical rotation deficits are noted mostly in upper cervical spine issues as in atlanto-axial joint pathology. Pain radiating to the occiput stems usually from C1 to C3 cervical pathology.[16]

Lower cervical spine pathology can manifest with axial pain (disc herniations, discogenic pain, lateral osteophyte formation and uncovertebral hypertrophy, cervical zygapophyseal joint hypertrophy). Neuropathic pain (radicular pain) affects most frequently the C6 and C7 nerve roots as a result of pathology at C5 to C6 and C6 to C7 vertebral levels. In a large prospective study conducted at Mayo Clinic for patients treated in a nonoperative fashion, although radicular pain had a high recurrence rate (31%), at a mean follow-up of 5.9 years, 90% of the patients experienced either mild pain or no pain.[17]

Significant Physical Examination Maneuvers for Patients with Neck Pain

If tandem walk (walking a line with 1 foot in front of the other) is normal, there is a low likelihood of cord compression or clinically significant spinal stenosis. This test can be used as a progression of disease measure. If the L'Hermitte sign (electrical-like sensations down spine or arms with passive flexion of neck) is present, one should suspect cervical myelopathy because this examination finding carries a greater than 90% specificity. A positive Spurling's maneuver (lateral flexion and rotation to the affected side with axial compression of the head reproducing radicular upper limb pain) is suggestive of cervical neuropathic pain/radiculitis with 85% to 95% specificity and 40% to 60% sensitivity.

Hoffmann's sign (involuntary flexion-adduction of thumb and index finger elicited with snapping flexion of the middle finger distal phalanx) is indicative of cervical myelopathy or demyelinating disorder with 50% to 80% sensitivity and 78% specificity. Neck distraction (relief of radicular upper limb symptoms when examiner grasps patient's head under occiput and chin and lifts, applying axial traction) indicates cervical radiculitis secondary to nerve compression with 90% specificity and up to 50% sensitivity. Upper limb strength testing should include assessment of hand grip, finger abduction, wrist extension, protonation and supination of the hand, flexion and extension at the elbow, and shoulder abduction. Deficits in strength may be indicative of myotomal weakness.

Sustained ankle clonus (>3 beats of clonus with constant brisk pressure on the sole of the forefoot) is significant for an upper motor neuron process such as demyelinating disease versus spinal cord compression versus spinal cord injury. Shoulder abduction, also known as the Bakody's sign (relief of ipsilateral cervical radicular pain with placing of the affected arm on the head through abduction of the shoulder), indicates cervical radiculitis with up to 90% specificity with moderate reliability.[18]

Cervical facet joint pain correlates with poor ergonomics or a mechanism of flexion/extension injury. Depending on the affected level, the patient may present with a complaint of occipital or temporoparietal pain (cervicogenic headache) or upper back and shoulder pain. Although examination findings may help to decrease suspicion of other possible causes of neck pain and shoulder pain, there is no physical examination maneuver to identify cervical facet joint pain. Imaging for cervical facet joint pain has not proven to help with diagnosis. Particularly after a whiplash injury, cervical facet joint pain can exist without evidence of discrete facet disease on MRI or CT scans. The diagnosis of cervical facet joint pain is well-established through controlled fluoroscopically guided contrast-enhanced diagnostic blocks for cases where neck pain did not resolve in a timely fashion (according to natural history).[19,20]

Diagnostic Workup

In patients with trauma to the head or neck, the NEXUS criteria and/or the Canadian C-spine criteria should be used to determine the need for further imaging.[14,15] History and physical examination along with risk factors should dictate further needs for imaging. Cervical spine radiographs with included flexion and extension views can determine instability (more than 3 mm difference in alignment between flexion and extensions views) in cervical spine segments. One recent study done in a surgical practice showed no change in clinical management based on the radiographic studies alone.[21]

CT scans of the cervical spine is rarely indicated in the absence of trauma and absence of prior surgery in the neck region. MRI is the most sensitive imaging modality for soft tissues structures (spinal cord, intervertebral disc, synovial cysts) and acute/subacute fractures. MRI is the only modality that can determine the acuity of a fracture. MRI should be considered in patients with red flag signs, progressive neurologic deficits, and for presurgical or preprocedural evaluation. Given the high rate of radiologic abnormalities in asymptomatic individuals,[22,23] caution should be exerted by the physician when ordering MRIs for chronic neck pain that does not respond to conservative treatment, in patients without red flag signs or neurologic deficits.

Electrodiagnostic studies constitute an extension of the physical examination. They should be used if there is a lack of correlation between physical examination and MRI, and to differentiate among cervical radiculopathy, peripheral nerve entrapment in the upper limb (neuropathy), and brachial plexopathy. In cases of weakness in any myotomal or nonmyotomal distribution, a physiatrist or a neurologist with electrodiagnostic skills should be consulted.[24]

Laboratory studies are not essential for evaluating musculoskeletal neck pain, unless other causes of neck pain are suspected (eg, rheumatologic disorder, infection, malignancy), in which case a complete blood count, erythrocyte sedimentation rate, and C-reactive protein might be an appropriate panel to send as a screening laboratory tool.

Treatment

Any clinician who is treating neck pain with or without radiation should be aware of the natural history of musculoskeletal neck pain.[17] In one randomized trial that followed 206 patients with acute cervical radicular pain, physical therapy, a home exercise program, and use of a hard collar significantly improved disability related to pain at 6 weeks compared with expectant ("wait and see") treatment.[25] Although there is no singular exercise modality for neck pain, a small prospective randomized trial demonstrated a trend toward greater improvement in the group that underwent the McKenzie Method of physical therapy compared with general exercise and expectant treatment. Patients may do well to work with a physical therapist trained to provide McKenzie physical therapy.[26]

The evidence for alternative treatments for neck pain including massage, acupuncture, manipulation, soft cervical collar, electrotherapy, and yoga being superior to sham or other treatments is weak. These treatments are equivalent to expectant treatment.[27–29] The evidence for pharmacologic interventions for acute and chronic musculoskeletal neck pain is limited. There are no high-quality studies to determine the efficacy of nonsteroidal anti-inflammatory drugs (NSAIDs) or oral steroids for neck pain. Cyclobenzaprine at doses of 15 or 30 mg/d was proven to be significantly more helpful than placebo for acute neck pain.[30]

Topical NSAID diclofenac etolamine 1.16% gel applied for acute neck pain was proven to be more helpful than placebo at 2 and 5 days after the start of treatment with 2 g of gel applied on the affected area up to four times daily. Efficacy assessments included pain on movement, pain at rest, functional neck disability index, and response to treatment (decrease in pain on movement by 50% after 48 hours). All measures achieved statistical significance.[31]

There is limited evidence for treatment of cervical musculoskeletal neck pain (in absence of clear cervical dystonia) with trigger point injections, dry needling, or botulinum toxin injections.[32–34] The combination treatment with a series of cervical epidural corticosteroid injections plus conservative treatment with adjuvants and physical therapy was superior to either treatment alone.[35] Of note, a systematic review and meta-analysis concluded that epidural local anesthetic and/or saline constituted an efficacious treatment, intermediate in efficacy between epidural corticosteroids and a true intramuscular placebo injection.[36]

In an era where the use of care and costs associated with the episode of care for cervical musculoskeletal neck pain have become paramount in maintaining access for the patient in need, the referring physician has the right to inquire about the number of epidural injections per year per new patient done by the interventionalist (injection performing physician) to achieve symptom management.

For cervical zygapophyseal joint pain confirmed through comparative fluoroscopically guided nerve blocks, fluoroscopically guided cervical medial branch radiofrequency heat neurotomy is effective for abolishing zygapophysial joint pain and carries only minor risks when performed according to Spine Intervention Society practice guidelines. The number of patients needed to treat for complete pain relief at 6 months is 2. The evidence of effectiveness is of high quality according to the GRADE system. The referring physician should have access to the outcome data and/or medication use in patients that receive radiofrequency ablation in a certain pain practice, to better select the best possible route for patient care.[37]

Spine surgery is rarely indicated for musculoskeletal axial neck pain. When neck pain is associated with progressive neurologic deficits or spinal cord compression, a surgical opinion is indicated. Patients with cervical radiculopathy might benefit in the short term from surgical decompression and/or fusion surgery. A randomized study that compared combined surgery and physical therapy with physical therapy alone for cervical radiculopathy found that surgery was associated with superior outcomes at 1 year, but by 2 years, the differences between groups were no longer statistically significant.[38]

The evidence for the use of biological therapies, including stem cell therapy, nerve growth factor, and cytokine inhibitors, is nonexistent for the treatment of musculoskeletal neck pain. Future research is needed to determine their efficacy for spinal pain and comparative effectiveness for all types of treatments including spinal surgeries, spine injection therapies and pharmacologic treatments.

Neck pain is the fourth leading cause of disability in the world. For patients with acute neck pain who receive appropriate treatment, most cases resolve over a period of weeks to months. Of note, a considerable proportion of individuals are left with residual or recurrent symptoms. History and physical examination may provide guidance on referral for advance imaging and/or spine surgery or specialist consultation. Clinical trials have found that physical therapy directed exercise programs may be beneficial, and for acute pain muscle relaxants are effective. There is good evidence for short-term relief ($\leq$4 weeks) to control radicular arm pain with cervical epidural steroid injections. In individuals with chronic axial pain secondary to zygapophyseal joint pathology, there is high-quality evidence in favor of radiofrequency denervation. More research studies are needed to compare efficacy, comparative effectiveness, and costs for neck pain treatment modalities, including spine surgeries, for specific defined cervical spine conditions.

LOWER BACK PAIN
Epidemiology

Lower back pain is the leading cause of disability and productivity loss worldwide with a lifetime prevalence of up to 84% for the adult patient population. The lifetime prevalence of lower back pain lasting at least 2 weeks is about 14%. The 6-month prevalence of disabling lower back pain is up to 11% of the adult patient population.[39,40] In 2010, lower back pain accounted for 1.3% of the diagnosis for an outpatient office visit.[41] The prevalence of activity limiting lower back pain that significantly interferes with work and quality of life for at least 1 day is 12%. One-month prevalence of lower back pain was estimated to be 20% to 26%.[42] Patients with acute lower back pain who present for medical care can have resolution of their symptoms in 70% to 90% of cases.[43,44] Although an acute episode may resolve, up to 70% of patients may suffer a recurrent episode of lower back pain within 1 year and 54% of them within 6 months. There is evidence that a prior episode of lower back pain has a fair predictive value for a future episode of lower back pain.[45,46]

Although it is not necessary to determine the benign causes for lower back pain, appropriate treatment for lower back pain conditions might decrease the chance for patients to develop chronic pain, a symptom that might be very difficult to reverse. In 1 recent large cohort study for the patients seen for acute lower back pain in the primary care setting, up to 20% of patients developed chronic lower back pain at the 2-year follow-up.[46]

A large study from Australia that followed 973 people with acute axial lower back pain seen in the primary care setting found that 28% did not fully recover 12 months after their initial consultation. Factors associated with persistence included older age, greater baseline pain and dysfunction, depression, fear of pain persistence, and continuing compensation claims.[47]

Although the number of studies that show significant change in the course of the disease by 1 visit to 1 specialist are limited, Fox and colleagues[48] show that a patient-centric approach to lower back pain can clearly improve outcomes and improve patient satisfaction while reducing the use of health care resources.

Patients who have at least 1 day of incapacitating lower back pain that interferes with life and work should see a primary care specialist for assessment of symptoms and counseling on ergonomics and activities. A consultation with a physical medicine and rehabilitation spine specialist within 48 hours for acute pain and within 10 days for all patients with lower back pain may significantly reduce further rate of surgical interventions and increase patients' satisfaction.[48] For patients who present to primary care, there is an approximately 4% incidence of vertebral compression fracture for patients more than 50 years old. The incidence for neoplastic disease of the spine is less than 0.1% for patients who obtain a study for lower back pain.[49]

Nontraumatic lower back pain can have different etiologies: intervertebral disc related, vertebral body related, facet joint related, and sacroiliac joint related. In addition, there are infectious, neoplasia (metastatic disease, lymphoma, myeloma, retroperitoneal tumors), and inflammatory arthropathies (ankylosing spondylitis, psoriatic arthritis) related lower back pain. Other causes that may mimic lumbar spine pathology can be related to renal disease (nephrolithiasis, renal capsule distension), pelvic organ pathology, aortic aneurysm or aortic pathology, or gastrointestinal disease (pancreatitis, gastroduodenal ulcer, etc). There are no high-quality heterogenous patient population studies on the natural history of subtypes of lower back and leg pain secondary to lumbar spine pathology based on anatomic pain generators.

Natural History

There is ample evidence that 28% to 65% of patients having 1 episode of axial back pain do not recover fully at 12 months after the initial consultation. Factors associated with ongoing pain included older age, greater baseline pain and dysfunction, depression, and fear of pain persistence.[46,47,50] Radicular lumbosacral pain has a similar natural history, with a better chance of improvement, up to 96% at 31 months.[51] However, a significant proportion (15%–40%) of patients can experience early (<1 year) or recurrent episodes of symptoms.[52] Radiologic studies show that approximately two-thirds of herniated lumbar discs undergo significant (>50%) resorption within 1 year, which can explain the natural history of radicular leg pain or lumbosacral radiculopathy.[53,54]

History and Physical Examination

In patients with lower back pain, there are few history and physical examination specific findings that would guide the treatment to a specific spinal procedure or surgery.

History

Lower back pain can be classified as acute (<4 weeks), subacute (4–12 weeks), or chronic (>12 weeks) regardless of the etiology. Lower back pain is a relatively rare manifestation of serious medical illness.[55] History elements should include any prior episode of the current pain, location of pain with patient pointing to the area of perceived pain, duration of symptoms, preferred relief positions and alleviating factors, and preferential direction (ie, movement of the lumbar spine or certain position/exercise abolishes or centralizes the radiating pain to the leg). It is also important to stratify the lower back pain as radicular (lower limb radiation) versus axial lower back pain (no radiation to the lower limbs), determine if patient had any recent falls, any gait abnormality, or bowel or bladder incontinence.

Physical examination

Focused physical examination can determine pathology that would require possible further specialty care:

- Toe walk and heel walk
- Use of assistive device
- Single leg raises on the toes ($\times$10 each)
- Single leg stands up from sitting position
- Weakness in manual muscle testing
- Pathologic reflexes, upper motor neuron signs, neurologic deficits (ankle clonus, Hoffman's, difficulty with tandem walk)
- Preferential direction of movement
- Segmental pain with spinous process percussion (compression fracture, metastatic disease to the spine)

Preferential direction of movement in patients with radicular or axial lower back pain symptoms can guide the patient's ergonomics and a physical therapy program, if there are no concerns for neurologic weakness. Physical therapy exercises matching the subjects' directional preference have been shown to significantly and rapidly decrease pain and medication use with improved outcomes.[56]

Myotomal weakness (leg weakness, foot drop, difficulty with balance) might be a good reason to refer to a spine nonoperative specialist for further evaluation, discussion of the prognosis of specific conditions, and discussion of the data in nonoperative and operative literature.

Minimal trauma in the elderly and other high-risk populations can result in a spinal compression fracture. The most sensitive examination findings are pain with forward flexion, pain with coughing or sneezing, and pain with percussion over the spinous processes. The patients can sometimes have a burst fracture that requires spine surgical consultation. This should be suspected if physical examination findings point to neurologic deficits.

The risk of developing lower back pain does not seem to be influenced by weight loss, smoking cessation, lumbar support (bracing), or chiropractic manipulations.[57,58]

Musculoskeletal Causes of Lower Back Pain

Discogenic pain can be the cause of lower back pain in patients with vascular ingrowth into the disc, disc uncovering due to spondylolisthesis, or exposure of disc nerve endings to inflammatory mediators. Disc-related pain is often worsened by activities like lifting, twisting, bending forward, and a history of sitting intolerance with improvement of pain with recumbency or standing.[59]

Herniated intervertebral disc refers to the anatomy of the disc on a MRI or CT scan. With contact or compression of nearby neural structures, a herniated intervertebral disc can manifest with radiation to the lower limb, in a dermatomal pattern with or without myotome weakness, also referred to as lumbar radiculopathy. The natural history of lumbar radiculopathy is favorable in most patients. Myotome weakness should trigger a consultation to a spine specialist who can further assess the deficit using electrodiagnostic studies (nerve conduction studies). The extreme case of a lumbar disc herniation can result in severe central stenosis with compression of the cauda equina resulting in bilateral leg pain, weakness, bladder dysfunction, and changes in perineal sensation. Cauda equina symptoms require emergent spine surgical evaluation.[60]

Lumbar zygapophyseal (facet) joint pain can be the cause for lower back pain especially in the setting of degenerative disc disease[61] or in the setting of severe degeneration of the zygapophyseal joint cartilage, presence of inflammatory cells and mediators, increased vascularization, and subchondral remodeling. This may contribute to spinal stenosis pathology.[62] Despite numerous attempts to use physical examination maneuvers to identify zygapophyseal joint pain, it was established that only diagnostic fluoroscopically guided contrast-enhanced blocks of the nerves that innervate the facet joints can accurately identify the pain generator.[63,64] Another etiology for axial lower back pain can be identified as a pars interarticularis defect which is called spondylolysis and can lead to spondylolisthesis (slip of the adjacent vertebra).[65]

Another cause of musculoskeletal lower back pain can be sacroiliac joint pain that occurs as a result of sacroiliitis, falls, or motor vehicle collisions.[66] Lumbar spinal stenosis can be associated with lower back pain and radicular limb pain. The radicular pain is provoked by standing and walking and immediately improved with sitting (83% specificity).[67,68] Lumbar spinal stenosis can be identified clinically with positive "shopping cart sign" (relief with leaning forward pushing a shopping cart).[69]

When to refer to a rehabilitation spine specialist or spine surgeon
- New back pain for patients who are 65 years or older.
- Back pain that does not improve within 4 to 5 weeks.
- Pain spreading into the lower leg, particularly if accompanied by weakness of the leg.
- Back pain as a result of falling or an accident, especially if patients are greater than 50 years of age.
- Pain that does not go away, even at night or when lying down.

When to refer to a spine surgeon or consider emergency room referral
- Urgent evaluation for symptomatology that uncovers weakness in 1 or both legs or problems with bladder, bowel, or sexual dysfunction, which can be signs of

cauda equina syndrome, arising from compression of the nerve bundle at the base of the spine.
- Back pain accompanied by unexplained fever or weight loss.
- A history of lower back pain associated with prior history of cancer, a weakened immune system, osteoporosis, or the use of corticosteroids for a prolonged period of time.

Tests

Laboratory tests might or might not increase suspicion for a systemic cause for lower back pain like inflammatory state, infection etiology, or tumor. A basic screen can include an erythrocyte sedimentation rate, C-reactive protein, and complete blood count.

Radiographs can be helpful to identify cortical bone defects including fractures, pars defect, or instability of the spine. In cases of instability or significant spondylolisthesis (one of the vertebrae of the lower spine slips forward in relation to another), it is reasonable to refer to a spine specialist.

MRI and CT scan of the lumbar spine are useful to identify more significant abnormalities like tumors, spondylodiscitis, osteomyelitis, or in procedural or surgical planning. These imaging modalities may be indicated in case of unresolved lower back pain within 4 to 5 weeks. MRI is the best imaging modality to assess for soft tissue changes (disc herniation, spine cysts, discitis). MRI with and without contrast can differentiate between scar tissue from prior surgery from disc material.

Fluoroscopically guided contrast-enhanced diagnostic blocks performed according to Spine Intervention Society guidelines are specific and sensitive procedures to identify or rule out a musculoskeletal structure of the spine as a pain generator.[70]

Treatment

Natural history (expectant progress) is the evolution of an episode of lower back pain without medical intervention. The clinical course is the response of the lower back pain to medical treatment. For musculoskeletal nonspecific acute lower back pain, there is fair evidence for treatment with NSAIDs for up to 3 months.[71] Despite the wide use of NSAIDs one should consider its significant side effect profile, including cardiovascular events, new-onset atrial fibrillation, congestive heart failure, stroke, heart attack, and drug–drug interactions that can occur.[72,73]

There is good evidence for the use of muscle relaxers, especially non–habit-forming (cyclobenzaprine) for the treatment of acute lower back pain.[74] There is no proven superiority of opioids to NSAIDs and muscle relaxers for treatment of musculoskeletal axial lower back pain. There is similar efficacy of duloxetine compared with NSAIDs and muscle relaxers in treatment of lower back pain.[75]

When performed by highly skilled physicians according to the guidelines, radiofrequency denervation of the lumbar facet joints can provide pain relief for up to 58% of patients who were carefully diagnosed with comparative diagnostic blocks.[76] There is good evidence that directional preference used in physical therapy sessions can significantly improve the lower back and lower limb symptoms.[56]

For patients with radicular leg pain secondary to a lumbar disc herniation, transforaminal epidural steroid injections have been shown to be effective. Using criteria of reduction of pain of more than 50%, success rates across studies showed 63% (58%–68%) at 1 month, 74% (68%–80%) at 3 months, 64% (59%–69%) at 6 months, and 64% (57%–71%) at 1 year.[77]

The extensive array of physical modalities, behavioral treatments, and widely used physical modalities including massage, acupuncture, therapeutic ultrasound treatments, yoga, Pilates, manipulative spinal therapies are not supported by the same level of evidence as the aforementioned treatments. Any improvement may be due to the natural time line of recovery.[78–87]

The goals for treatment in patients with acute musculoskeletal lower back pain is to provide short-term symptom management. Nonpharmacologic treatment including mechanical diagnosis and treatment and avoiding bedrest are good first steps. Anti-inflammatory medications along with muscle relaxers can also be used. There is controversial literature for opioid treatment in acute musculoskeletal lower back pain.

Patient education is probably the most important aspect of the initial visit for acute lower back pain with or without radicular symptoms. There is ample evidence that seeing a nonoperative physiatry spine specialist within 1 week can increase patient satisfaction, decrease use of care and reduce rates of fusion spine surgeries for patients with lower back pain.[48]

DISCLOSURE

Nothing to disclose.

REFERENCES

1. Murray CJ, Atkinson C, Bhalla K, et al. The state of US health, 1990-2010: burden of diseases, injuries, and risk factors. JAMA 2013;310:591–608.
2. Badley EM, Tennant A. Changing profile of joint disorders with age: findings from a postal survey of the population of Calderdale, West Yorkshire, United Kingdom. Ann Rheum Dis 1992;51:366–71.
3. Cote P, Cassidy JD, Carroll L. The Saskatchewan health and back pain survey. The prevalence of neck pain and related disability in Saskatchewan adults. Spine 1998;23:1689–98.
4. Isacsson A, Hanson BS, Ranstam J, et al. Social network, social support and the prevalence of neck and low back pain after retirement. A population study of men born in 1914 in Malmo, Sweden. Scand J Soc Med 1995;23:17–22.
5. Brochet B, Michel P, Barberger-Gateau P, et al. Population-based study of pain in elderly people: a descriptive survey. Age Ageing 1998;27:279–84.
6. Woo J, Ho SC, Lau J, et al. Musculoskeletal complaints and associated consequences in elderly Chinese aged 70 years and over. J Rheumatol 1994;21: 1927–31.
7. Fejer R, Kyvik KO, Hartvigsen J. The prevalence of neck pain in the world population: a systematic critical review of the literature. Eur Spine J 2006;15:834–48.
8. Cohen SP, Hooten WM. Advances in the diagnosis and management of neck pain [review]. BMJ 2017;358:j3221.
9. May S, Gardiner E, Young S, et al. Predictor variables for a positive long-term functional outcome in patients with acute and chronic neck and back pain treated with a McKenzie approach: a secondary analysis. J Man Manip Ther 2008;16: 155–60.
10. Peterson C, Bolton J, Humphreys BK. Predictors of outcome in neck pain patients undergoing chiropractic care: comparison of acute and chronic patients. Chiropr Man Ther 2012;20:27.
11. Vasseljen O, Woodhouse A, Bjørngaard JH, et al. Natural course of acute neck and low back pain in the general population: the HUNT study. Pain 2013;154: 1237–44.

12. Vos CJ, Verhagen AP, Passchier J, et al. Clinical course and prognostic factors in acute neck pain: an inception cohort study in general practice. Pain Med 2008;9: 572–80.
13. Christensen JO, Knardahl S. Time-course of occupational psychological and social factors as predictors of new-onset and persistent neck pain: a three-wave prospective study over 4 years. Pain 2014;155:1262–71.
14. Stiell IG, Wells GA, Vandemheen KL, et al. The Canadian C-spine rule for radiography in alert and stable trauma patients. JAMA 2001;286(15):1841–8.
15. Hoffman JR, Mower WR, Wolfson AB, et al. Validity of a set of clinical criteria to rule out injury to the cervical spine in patients with blunt trauma. National Emergency X-Radiography Utilization Study Group. N Engl J Med 2000;343(2):94–9 [Erratum appears in N Engl J Med 2001;344(6):464].
16. Dreyfuss P, Michaelsen M, Fletcher D. Atlanto-occipital and lateral atlanto-axial joint pain patterns. Spine (Phila Pa 1976) 1994;19:1125–31.
17. Radhakrishnan K, Litchy WJ, O'Fallon WM, et al. Epidemiology of cervical radiculopathy: a population-based study from Rochester, Minnesota, 1976 through 1990. Brain 1994;117:325–35.
18. Rubinstein SM, Pool JJ, van Tulder MW, et al. A systematic review of the diagnostic accuracy of provocative tests of the neck for diagnosing cervical radiculopathy. Eur Spine J 2007;16:307–19.
19. Barnsley L, Bogduk N. Medial branch blocks are specific for the diagnosis of cervical zygapophyseal joint pain. Reg Anesth 1993;18(6):343.
20. Barnsley L, Lord S, Bogduk N. Comparative local anaesthetic blocks in the diagnosis of cervical zygapophysial joint pain. Pain 1993;55(1):99.
21. White AP, Biswas D, Smart LR, et al. Utility of flexion-extension radiographs in evaluating the degenerative cervical spine. Spine (Phila Pa 1976) 2007; 32(9):975.
22. Matsumoto M, Fujimura Y, Suzuki N, et al. MRI of cervical intervertebral discs in asymptomatic subjects. J Bone Joint Surg Br 1998;80:19–24.
23. Lehto IJ, Tertti MO, Komu ME, et al. Age-related MRI changes at 0.1 T in cervical discs in asymptomatic subjects. Neuroradiology 1994;36:49–53.
24. Dillingham TR, Lauder TD, Andary M, et al. Identification of cervical radiculopathies: optimizing the electromyographic screen. Am J Phys Med Rehabil 2001; 80(2):84–91.
25. Kuijper B, Tans JT, Beelen A, et al. Cervical collar or physiotherapy versus wait and see policy for recent onset cervical radiculopathy: randomised trial. BMJ 2009;339:b3883.
26. Kjellman G, Oberg B. A randomized clinical trial comparing general exercise, McKenzie treatment and a control group in patients with neck pain. J Rehabil Med 2002;34(4):183–90.
27. Thoomes EJ, Scholten-Peeters W, Koes B, et al. The effectiveness of conservative treatment for patients with cervical radiculopathy: a systematic review. Clin J Pain 2013;29:1073–86.
28. Kong LJ, Zhan HS, Cheng YW, et al. Massage therapy for neck and shoulder pain: a systematic review and meta-analysis. Evid Based Complement Alternat Med 2013;2013:613279.
29. Patel KC, Gross A, Graham N, et al. Massage for mechanical neck disorders. Cochrane Database Syst Rev 2012;(9):CD004871.
30. Borenstein DG, Korn S. Efficacy of a low-dose regimen of cyclobenzaprine hydrochloride in acute skeletal muscle spasm: results of two placebo-controlled trials. Clin Ther 2003;25:1056–73.

31. Predel HG, Giannetti B, Pabst H, et al. Efficacy and safety of diclofenac diethyl-amine 1.16% gel in acute neck pain: a randomized, double-blind, placebo-controlled study. BMC Musculoskelet Disord 2013;14:250.

32. Scott NA, Guo B, Barton PM, et al. Trigger point injections for chronic non-malignant musculoskeletal pain: a systematic review. Pain Med 2009;10:54–69.

33. Kamanli A, Kaya A, Ardicoglu O, et al. Comparison of lidocaine injection, botuli-num toxin injection, and dry needling to trigger points in myofascial pain syn-drome. Rheumatol Int 2005;25:604–11.

34. Qerama E, Fuglsang-Frederiksen A, Kasch H, et al. A double-blind, controlled study of botulinum toxin A in chronic myofascial pain. Neurology 2006;67:241–5.

35. Cohen SP, Hayek S, Semenov Y, et al. Epidural steroid injections, conservative treatment or combination treatment for cervical radiculopathy: a multi-center, ran-domized, comparative-effectiveness study. Anesthesiology 2014;121:1045–55.

36. Bicket MC, Gupta A, Brown CH, et al. Epidural injections for spinal pain: a sys-tematic review and meta-analysis evaluating the "control" injections in random-ized controlled trials. Anesthesiology 2013;119:907–31.

37. Engel A, Rappard G, King W, et al, Standards Division of the International Spine Intervention Society. The effectiveness and risks of fluoroscopically-guided cervi-cal medial branch thermal radiofrequency neurotomy: a systematic review with comprehensive analysis of the published data [review]. Pain Med 2016;17(4):658–69.

38. Engquist M, Löfgren H, Öberg B, et al. Surgery versus nonsurgical treatment of cervical radiculopathy: a prospective, randomized study comparing surgery plus physiotherapy with physiotherapy alone with a 2-year follow-up. Spine (Phila Pa 1976) 2013;38:1715–22.

39. Deyo RA, Tsui-Wu YJ. Descriptive epidemiology of low-back pain and its related medical care in the United States. Spine (Phila Pa 1976) 1987;12(3):264.

40. Cassidy JD, Carroll LJ. Côté Saskatchewan health and back pain survey. The prevalence of low back pain and related disability in Saskatchewan adults. Spine (Phila Pa 1976) 1998;23(17):1860.

41. Centers for Disease Control and Prevention. National Ambulatory Medical Care Survey: 2010 Summary Tables. Available at: http://www.cdc.gov/nchs/data/ahcd/namcs_summary/2010_namcs_web_tables.pdf. Accessed September 30, 2014.

42. Hoy D, Bain C, Williams G, et al. A systematic review of the global prevalence of low back pain. Arthritis Rheum 2012;64(6):2028–37.

43. Coste J, Delecoeuillerie G, Cohen de Lara A, et al. Clinical course and prognostic factors in acute low back pain: an inception cohort study in primary care practice. BMJ 1994;308(6928):577.

44. Cherkin DC, Deyo RA, Street JH, et al. Predicting poor outcomes for back pain seen in primary care using patients' own criteria. Spine (Phila Pa 1976) 1996;21(24):2900.

45. Pengel LH, Herbert RD, Maher CG, et al. Acute low back pain: systematic review of its prognosis. BMJ 2003;327(7410):323.

46. Mehling WE, Gopisetty V, Bartmess E, et al. The prognosis of acute low back pain in primary care in the United States: a 2-year prospective cohort study. Spine (Phila Pa 1976) 2012;37(8):678–84.

47. Henschke N, Maher CG, Refshauge KM, et al. Prognosis in patients with recent onset low back pain in Australian primary care: inception cohort study. BMJ 2008;337:a171.

48. Fox J, Haig AJ, Todey B, et al. The effect of required physiatrist consultation on surgery rates for back pain. Spine (Phila Pa 1976) 2013;38(3):E178–84.
49. Jarvik JG, Deyo RA. Diagnostic evaluation of low back pain with emphasis on imaging [review]. Ann Intern Med 2002;137(7):586–97.
50. Itz CJ, Geurts JW, van Kleef M, et al. Clinical course of non-specific low back pain: a systematic review of prospective cohort studies set in primary care. Eur J Pain 2013;17:5–15.
51. Saal JA, Saal JS. Nonoperative treatment of herniated lumbar intervertebral disc with radiculopathy: an outcome study. Spine (Phila Pa 1976) 1989;14:431–7.
52. Suri P, Rainville J, Hunter DJ, et al. Recurrence of radicular pain or back pain after nonsurgical treatment of symptomatic lumbar disk herniation. Arch Phys Med Rehabil 2012;93:690–5.
53. Saal JA. Natural history and nonoperative treatment of lumbar disc herniation. Spine (Phila Pa 1976) 1996;21:2S–9S.
54. Benoist M. The natural history of lumbar disc herniation and radiculopathy. Joint Bone Spine 2002;69:155–60.
55. Chou R. In the clinic. Low back pain. Ann Intern Med 2014;160(11). ITC6-1.
56. Long A, Donelson R, Fung T. Does it matter which exercise? A randomized control trial of exercise for low back pain. Spine (Phila Pa 1976) 2004;29(23): 2593–602.
57. Lahad A, Malter AD, Berg AO, et al. JAMA 1994;272(16):1286.
58. Cherkin DC, Deyo RA, Battié M, et al. A comparison of physical therapy, chiropractic manipulation, and provision of an educational booklet for the treatment of patients with low back pain. N Engl J Med 1998;339(15):1021.
59. Simon J, McAuliffe M, Shamim F, et al. Discogenic low back pain. Phys Med Rehabil Clin N Am 2014;25:305–17.
60. Gardner A, Gardner E, Morley T. Cauda equina syndrome: a review of the current clinical and medico-legal position. Eur Spine J 2011;20:690–7.
61. Yang KH, King AI. Mechanism of facet load transmission as a hypothesis for low-back pain. Spine (Phila Pa 1976) 1984;9:557–65.
62. Izzo R, Guarnieri G, Guglielmi G, et al. Biomechanics of the spine. Part I: spinal stability. Eur J Radiol 2013;82:118–26.
63. Schwarzer AC, Aprill CN, Derby R, et al. Clinical features of patients with pain stemming from the lumbar zygapophysial joints: is the lumbar facet syndrome a clinical entity? Spine (Phila Pa 1976) 1994;19:1132–7.
64. Laslett M, McDonald B, Aprill CN, et al. Clinical predictors of screening lumbar zygapophyseal joint blocks: development of clinical prediction rules. Spine J 2006;6:370–9.
65. Leone A, Cianfoni A, Cerase A, et al. Lumbar spondylolysis: a review. Skeletal Radiol 2011;40:683–700.
66. Cohen SP, Chen Y, Neufeld NJ. Sacroiliac joint pain: a comprehensive review of epidemiology, diagnosis and treatment. Expert Rev Neurother 2013;13:99–116.
67. Katz JN, Dalgas M, Stucki G, et al. Degenerative lumbar spinal stenosis. Diagnostic value of the history and physical examination. Arthritis Rheum 1995;38: 1236–41.
68. Suri P, Rainville J, Kalichman L, et al. Does this older adult with lower extremity pain have the clinical syndrome of lumbar spinal stenosis? JAMA 2010;304: 2628–36.
69. Nadeau M, Rosas-Arellano MP, Gurr KR, et al. The reliability of differentiating neurogenic claudication from vascular claudication based on symptomatic presentation. Can J Surg 2013;56:372–7.

70. Curatolo M, Bogduk N. Diagnostic blocks for chronic pain. Scand J Pain 2010; 1(4):186–92.
71. Kuijpers T, van Middelkoop M, Rubinstein SM, et al. A systematic review on the effectiveness of pharmacological interventions for chronic non-specific low-back pain. Eur Spine J 2011;20:40–50.
72. Schmidt M, Lamberts M, Olsen AM, et al. Cardiovascular safety of non-aspirin non-steroidal anti-inflammatory drugs: review and position paper by the working group for Cardiovascular Pharmacotherapy of the European Society of Cardiology [review]. Eur Heart J 2016;37(13):1015–23.
73. Schmidt M, Christiansen CF, Mehnert F, et al. Non-steroidal anti-inflammatory drug use and risk of atrial fibrillation or flutter: population based case-control study. BMJ 2011;343:d3450.
74. van Tulder MW, Touray T, Furlan AD, et al. Muscle relaxants for nonspecific low back pain: a systematic review within the framework of the Cochrane collaboration. Spine (Phila Pa 1976) 2003;28:1978–92.
75. Cawston H, Davie A, Paget MA, et al. Efficacy of duloxetine versus alternative oral therapies: an indirect comparison of randomised clinical trials in chronic low back pain. Eur Spine J 2013;22:1996–2009.
76. MacVicar J, Borowczyk JM, MacVicar AM, et al. Lumbar medial branch radiofrequency neurotomy in New Zealand. Pain Med 2013;14(5):639–45.
77. Smith CC, McCormick ZL, Mattie R, et al. The effectiveness of lumbar transforaminal injection of steroid for the treatment of radicular pain: a comprehensive review of the published data. Pain Med 2019. https://doi.org/10.1093/pm/pnz160 [pii:pnz160].
78. Wells C, Kolt GS, Marshall P, et al. The effectiveness of Pilates exercise in people with chronic low back pain: a systematic review. PLoS One 2014;9:e100402.
79. Cramer H, Lauche R, Haller H, et al. A systematic review and meta-analysis of yoga for low back pain. Clin J Pain 2013;29:450–60.
80. Kizhakkeveettil A, Rose K, Kadar GE. Integrative therapies for low back pain that include complementary and alternative medicine care: a systematic review. Glob Adv Health Med 2014;3:49–64.
81. Ebadi S, Henschke N, Nakhostin Ansari N, et al. Therapeutic ultrasound for chronic low-back pain. Cochrane Database Syst Rev 2014;(3):CD009169.
82. Franke H, Franke JD, Fryer G. Osteopathic manipulative treatment for nonspecific low back pain: a systematic review and meta-analysis. BMC Musculoskelet Disord 2014;15:286.
83. Slade SC, Patel S, Underwood M, et al. What are patient beliefs and perceptions about exercise for nonspecific chronic low back pain? A systematic review of qualitative studies. Clin J Pain 2014;30:995–1005.
84. Furlan AD, Imamura M, Dryden T, et al. Massage for low back pain: an updated systematic review within the framework of the Cochrane Back Review Group. Spine (Phila Pa 1976) 2009;34:1669–84.
85. Lam M, Galvin R, Curry P. Effectiveness of acupuncture for nonspecific chronic low back pain: a systematic review and meta-analysis. Spine (Phila Pa 1976) 2013;38:2124–38.
86. Franke H, Fryer G, Ostelo RW, et al. Muscle energy technique for non-specific low-back pain. Cochrane Database Syst Rev 2015;(2):CD009852.
87. Rubinstein SM, van Middelkoop M, Kuijpers T, et al. A systematic review on the effectiveness of complementary and alternative medicine for chronic non-specific low-back pain. Eur Spine J 2010;19:1213–28.

Osteoarthritis
Pathology, Diagnosis, and Treatment Options

Benjamin Abramoff, MD, MS, Franklin E. Caldera, DO, MBA*

KEYWORDS

- Osteoarthritis • Arthralgia • Arthritis • Degenerative joint disease

KEY POINTS

- There are many modifiable and nonmodifiable risk factors for osteoarthritis (OA): genetic predisposition, increasing age, obesity, metabolic syndrome, previous injury, lifestyle factors, and female gender.
- Progressive pain is the most prominent symptom in OA, although mechanical symptoms may also be present. Systemic symptoms should be absent and their presence should cause investigation into other pathologies.
- Plain radiographs, diagnostic ultrasound, and MRI are tools that can help diagnose OA and guide treatment recommendations. Radiographic findings include joint space narrowing, osteophytosis, subchondral sclerosis, and cyst formation.
- Traditional treatment options include lifestyle modification, physical therapy, oral medications, injections, physical modalities, and surgery. Numerous novel treatments are being investigated, such as nerve blocks, mesenchymal stem cell injections, platelet-rich plasma injections, and strontium ranelate.

INTRODUCTION

Osteoarthritis (OA) is endemic throughout the world. An estimated 30.8 million adults in the United States and 300 million individuals worldwide are living with OA.[1,2] It is the leading cause of disability in older adults and leads to pain, loss of function, and decreased quality of life (QOL).[3,4]

On a societal scale, OA is estimated to cost $303 billion dollars annually in medical costs and lost earnings.[5] Continued efforts are needed to reduce the occurrence, pain, and loss of function from this chronic, debilitating disease. This article is a review of OA—pathology, diagnosis, and treatment options.

Department of PM&R, University of Pennsylvania, Penn Medicine Rittenhouse, 1800 Lombard Street, Philadelphia, PA 19146, USA
* Corresponding author.
E-mail address: Franklin.caldera@uphs.upenn.edu

Med Clin N Am 104 (2020) 293–311
https://doi.org/10.1016/j.mcna.2019.10.007
0025-7125/20/© 2019 Elsevier Inc. All rights reserved.

medical.theclinics.com

PATHOLOGY

Previously, OA was thought to be a simply a disease of "wear and tear." Chronic overload and impaired biomechanics on the joint were thought to lead to destruction of the joint's articular cartilage and resultant inflammation. This subsequently led to stiffness, swelling, and loss of mobility. It is now known that OA is a much more complex process composed of inflammatory and metabolic factors.[6,7]

OA is most notable for its effect on articular cartilage, which gets severely degraded over the course of the disease. Articular cartilage is the smooth cartilage at the end of long bones and within the intervertebral discs. It provides a low friction surface for articulation while being able to transmit heavy loads. Although the half-life of the collagen within the cartilage is long, it heals very slowly if at all, even with minor injuries. Although the cartilage has the most notable changes, the entire joint is affected, including the synovium, joint ligaments, and subchondral bone.[7]

Inflammation including active synovitis and systemic inflammation play a key role in the pathogenesis of OA. One potential explanation is that degraded cartilage induces a foreign body reaction within the synovial cells. This may lead to production of metalloproteases, synovial angiogenesis, and production of inflammatory cytokines, which leads to further cartilage destruction. Other theories propose a central role of activated synovial macrophages and the innate immune system in the progression of OA.[8]

Systemic inflammation may also play a role in the pathogenesis of OA. A study by Yusuf and colleagues[9] (2010) found that body weight was a strong risk factor for developing hand OA. This suggests other consequences of obesity may be at play beyond body-weight and joint mechanics. This study and others suggest that systemic factors related to obesity, metabolic syndrome, and atherosclerosis likely play a systemic role in the development of OA, possibly through leptin and other adipokines. Direct effects of aging on cartilage (due to chondrocyte senescence, DNA damage, aging of the cartilage matrix, oxidative stress, mitochondrial dysfunction, and autophagy) as well as the effect of the endocrine system and estrogen on joint health are also being investigated.[8,10]

RISK FACTORS

OA is a complex disease with many elements that potentially may lead to its presentation and progression (**Fig. 1**). OA can be broadly classified into 2 types:

Primary OA—no known cause
Secondary OA—caused by other conditions such as trauma, obesity, or disease

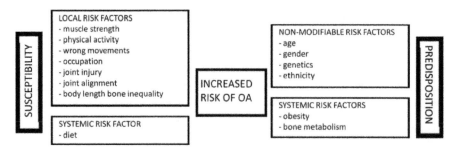

Fig. 1. Risk factors that lead to the development of OA. (*From* Musumeci G, Aiello FC., Szychlinska MA, et al. Osteoarthritis in the XXIst century: Risk factors and behaviours that influence disease onset and progression. Int J Mol Sci 2015;16(3):6096; with permission.)

This section discusses some of the known modifiable and nonmodifiable risk factors for OA.

Age

Although prevalence numbers vary, particularly due to varying definitions of OA, it is conclusive that aging is the single greatest risk factor for the development of OA. The presence of both radiographic and symptomatic OA increases over the human lifespan. Increased rates with aging have been noted in the knee, hip, and hand.[11] Worldwide estimates are that 9.6% of men and 18% of women older than 60 years have symptomatic OA.[12] The Framingham Osteoarthritis study found that 27% of those aged 63 to 70 years had radiographic evidence of knee OA, increasing to 44% in the age group older than 80 years.[13]

Genetic and Epigenetic Predisposition

Susceptibility to OA is considered polygenetic in nature; there are more than 80 genes that have been implicated in the pathogenesis. Some of these genes are for vitamin D receptors and insulin-like growth factor 1. OA has also been associated with a single-nucleotide polymorphism in the growth and differentiation factor 5 gene, which is involved in the development of healthy bone and cartilage.[6] Epigenetic mechanisms including DNA methylation, histone modification, and microRNAs are currently being investigated for their role in the development of OA.[14]

Obesity/Metabolic Syndrome

Obesity and metabolic syndrome are also strong risk factors for the development of OA. A meta-analysis found that the odds ratio (OR) for having OA in obese or over-weight individuals compared with normal-weight individuals was 2.96.[15] Evidence is accumulating that prove that dyslipidemia and type 2 diabetes are risk factors for OA independent of obesity.[16]

Endocrine

There is a 3 times higher risk of progression of knee OA in patients with low levels of vitamin C or D.[13] Despite being postulated, increasing bone density has not been shown to lead to increased risk of OA.[17]

Gender

Most studies suggest that women are more likely to develop symptomatic knee problems compared with men (with analysis demonstrating a pooled OR of 1.84).[15] A large study of Spanish patients by Prieto-Alhambra and colleagues[18] (2013) found that the relative risk of OA in the hands, knee, and hip were 1.52 times greater in women than in men. This difference was more pronounced in the hip/hand (relative risk [RR] 2.50) compared with the knee (RR 1.19). These differences peaked at 70 to 75 years of age for the knee and hip. Interestingly, the sex difference for hand OA peaked at 50 to 55 years of age. Despite this overall trend, OA is more prevalent in men than women under the age of 50 years. This prevalence changes over the age of 50 years where OA risk is higher in women than men.[13]

Previous Injury

Posttraumatic OA may be caused by any inciting event leading to damage to the joint, including fractures, cartilage damage, ligamentous injury, or meniscal injuries. A 2006 study by Brown and colleagues[19] estimated that 12% of all OA is posttraumatic in nature. Prevalence of previous injury varies by joint; posttraumatic OA accounts for 20% to 78% of cases of ankle OA, 10% of knee OA, and 2% of hip OA.[20]

Occupation

There is some evidence that excessive kneeling, squatting, jumping, bending, and lifting can lead to knee OA.[21,22] Construction workers, forestry workers, and farmers have been found to be at particular high risk.[23] Military populations also have been found to have much higher rates of OA than the general population.[24]

An association between the increasing use of technology, computers, and smartphones and hand OA has yet to be proved but is a common concern that requires further investigation, as these technologies have become increasingly prevalent in our lives.[6]

Sports

Joint degeneration can also occur in athletes and younger individuals through damage to the articular cartilage from repetitive impact and loading. Sports like football and soccer account for the most impact damage secondary to direct blunt trauma. It has been shown that more than 80% of American football players with a history of knee injuries had evidence of OA 10 to 30 years after competing.[25]

Ethnicity

There is some evidence that race and ethnicity play a role in the prevalence of OA in different populations. OA is more common in Europeans than in Asians, Africans, and Jamaicans.[13] Also, OA is more prevalent in Europe and the United States than in other parts of the world.[26] There may even be differences between joints, for example, there is evidence that Chinese individuals may have lower risk for hand and hip OA while concurrently having a higher risk of knee OA. Severity, gender predication, and specific OA features may also differ by ethnicity.[27]

Joint Shape and Dysplasia

Congenital abnormalities of joints, such as acetabular dysplasia, slipped capital femoral epiphysis, hallux valgus, and valgus/valgus joint alignment likely play a role in the development and progression of OA.[27,28]

SYMPTOMS

Pain is the most prominent symptom in patients with OA. A 2008 study by Hawker and colleagues of the pain experience of those with OA found that pain tends to come in 2 forms, a constant background aching pain and intermittent intense pain. Pain with OA is also noted to slowly and insidiously progress with time. Early in the course, the pain is predictable and caused by specific (often high-impact) activities. Over time, pain and other joint symptoms become less predictable and more constant, with daily activities beginning to become affected. In advanced stages, constant dull and aching pain is accompanied by unpredictable, intense, severe pain, which leads to avoidance of certain activities.[29] A full list of patient-reported symptoms and their frequency are noted in **Table 1**.

It is worth noting that the degree of structural pathology noted on imaging and the degree of pain are not always concordant with the symptoms of OA. Some individuals with severe pain have a paucity of findings on imaging and vice versa. Elements such as prior pain experiences, treatment expectations, psychological factors, and sociocultural environment all potentially play a role in the individual's experience of pain.[30]

Table 1
Frequency of pain complaints in osteoarthritis

Rank	Feature	Frequency N (%)	Distress (/6) Mean ± SD (Range)	Points (/10) Mean ± SD (Range)
1	Sharp pain	65 (71.4)	4.2 ± 1.4 (1–6)	2.8 ± 2.1 (0–9)
2	Limitation of activities	63 (69.2)	4.1 ± 1.3. (0–6)	2.6 ± 2.1 (0–10)
3	Ache/dull	60 (65.9)	3.6 ± 1.6 (0–6)	2.4 ± 2.1 (0–10)
4	Triggered by activity	46 (50.5)	4.2 ± 1.3 (1–6)	3.0 ± 2.1 (0–10)
5	Stiffness	24 (26.4)	4.0 ± 1.2 (2–6)	2.9 ± 2.7 (0–10)
6	Unpredictability	23 (25.3)	3.4 ± 1.6 (1–6)	1.4 ± 1.5 (0–6)
7	Constant	21 (23.1)	3.9 ± 1.5 (1–6)	2.1 ± 1.4 (0–5)
8	Unstable	20 (22.0)	4.3 ± 1.6 (1–6)	2.2 ± 1.5 (0–5)
9	Night pain/impact on sleep	16 (17.6)	3.9 ± 1.4 (1–6)	2.9 ± 1.4 (1–5)
10	Mood	16 (17.6)	3.8 ± 1.5 (1–6)	1.6 ± 1.7 (0–5)
11	Swelling	14 (15.4)	3.9 ± 1.8 (0–6)	1.6 ± 1.2 (0–4)
12	Grating	12 (13.2)	4.3 ± 1.3 (2–6)	1.8 ± 1.3 (0–4)
13	Inactivity	12 (13.2)	3.5 ± 1.2 (1–5)	2.0 ± 1.0 (0–3)
14	Burning pain	6 (6.6)	4.2 ± 2.3 (0–6)	3.7 ± 1.4 (2–6)
15	Weakness	6 (6.6)	2.5 ± 1.9 (0–5)	2.2 ± 0.8 (1–3)
16	Fear	6 (6.6)	4.0 ± 2.0 (L–6)	2.0 ± 1.7 (0–4)
17	Use of medication/devices	5 (5.5)	4.2 ± 1.3 (3–6)	1.4 ± 1.1 (0–3)
18	Numbness	4 (4.4)	3.5 ± 2.1 (1–6)	1.5 ± 1.9 (0–4)
19	Locking	4 (4.4)	4.5 ± 1.3 (3–6)	2.3 ± 1.3. (1–4)
20	Cramping/muscle spasms	3 (3.3)	4.7 ± 0.6 (4–5)	2.3 ± 2.3 (1–5)
21	Clicking/cracking	3 (33)	3.0 ± 0.0 (3)	2.0 ± 2.7 (0–5)
22	Radiating pain	1 (1.1)	6 (6)	1 (1)

From Hawker GA, Stewart L, French MR, et al. Understanding the pain experience in hip and knee osteoarthritis–an OARSI/OMERACT initiative. Osteoarthritis Cartilage 2008;16(4):420; with permission.

Other nonpain symptoms of OA include joint swelling, clicking, locking, grating, crepitus, cramping, reduced range of motion, and deformity. Also described are symptoms of instability, buckling, or "giving way." Patients with OA complain of morning stiffness that improves in 30 minutes. This is unlike in rheumatoid arthritis, which typically last longer. The pain of OA also increases throughout the day and with increased activity.

Systemic symptoms should be absent. This includes fever, weight loss, or abnormal blood test. The presence of such symptoms would alert the physician to other disease processes such as infection or malignancy.[31]

The symptoms of OA have been noted to lead to a loss of independence and impaired ability for individuals to do the activities that they enjoy.[29] A large study of 10,000 patients by Fautrel and colleagues (2005) found that 81.5% of patients with OA reported limitations in their activities of daily living; 61.1% reported limited mobility outside the home and 12.8% in the home (compared with 10.2% and 2.8% in the general population, respectively). Patients with OA also noted significantly more impairment that the general population in grocery shopping, house cleaning, and dressing. Leisure activities including sports and gardening were also significantly affected. Individuals with OA also missed more work compared with a control population.[32]

Overall, quality of life (QOL) is significantly affected by OA in multiple domains. Although clearly there is a diminished QOL in terms of physical functioning, adverse effects on mental health have been noted as well.[33]

EXAMINATION FINDINGS

Typical joints affected by OA include the knee, hip, distal and proximal interphalangeal joints, first trapeziometacarpal (carpometacarpal) joints, the first metatarsophalangeal joint, and the facet joints of the spine. Other joints including the elbow, wrist, shoulder, and ankle are less common.

There are many clinical features seen in patients with OA that may be due to synovial fluid accumulation, active inflammation, or bony deformity of the joints. Some common clinical findings include joint line tenderness, reduced range of both passive and active movement, crepitus, joint effusion, and bony swelling and deformity. These findings can be localized to one joint or polyarticular in nature. Heberden and Bouchard nodes (swelling at the distal and proximal interphalangeal joints, respectively) are also commonly noted.

The presence of a popliteal cyst is often the sequela of OA of the knee. One may also see valgus or varus deformity. In the hip, limited internal rotation is commonly seen on examination. Crepitus and decrease in range of motion, especially external rotation, is often seen on physical examination of the shoulder.

In OA of the foot, pain may be seen in the first metatarsophalangeal joint with limited range of motion of the first metatarsophalangeal joint. One may also see hallux valgus deformity on physical examination.

IMAGING

OA is primarily a clinical diagnosis. However, plain radiography can be helpful in confirming the diagnosis and ruling out other pathology.[34] MRI and computed tomography are rarely needed.

There are certain plain radiographic findings characteristic of OA. OA often demonstrates joint space narrowing, osteophyte formation, subchondral sclerosis, and cysts (**Figs. 2–5**).

The knee joint is typically evaluated by using extended knee radiographs, while the patient is weight bearing. Flexed knee radiographs are also used to improve intraarticular visualization. There are multiple grading schemes used for evaluation of joint space narrowing or osteophyte formation.[35] One of the most common grading schemes used in OA is the Kellgren-Lawrence classification system.

Radiographic features of OA described by Kellgren and Lawrence include evaluation of the following: formation of osteophytes on joint margins or on tibial spines, periarticular ossicles (distal or proximal interphalangeal joints), narrowing of joint cartilage associated with sclerosis of subchondral bone, small pseudocystic areas with sclerotic walls situated in the subchondral bone, and altered shape of bone ends, particularly in the head of the femur:

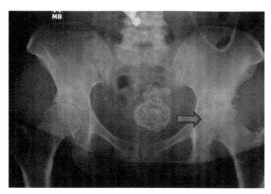

Fig. 2. Severe left narrowing of the hip joint space (*arrow*).

Grade 0: demonstrated no joint space narrowing or reactive changes.
Grade 1: doubtful joint space narrowing, possible osteophytic lipping.
Grade 2: definitive osteophytes, possible joint space narrowing.
Grade 3: moderate osteophytes, definite joint space narrowing and possible bone end deformity.
Grade 4: large osteophytes, marked joint space narrowing, severe sclerosis, definite bone end deformity.[36]

Recently, additional modalities such as MRI, ultrasound, and optical coherence tomography have enhanced OA diagnosis and management.

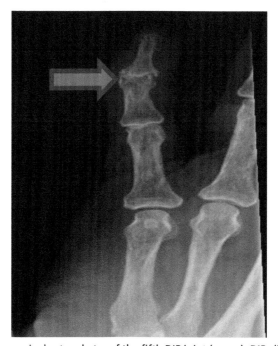

Fig. 3. Moderate marginal osteophytes of the fifth DIP joint (*arrow*). DIP, distal interphalangeal joint.

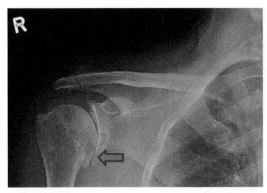

Fig. 4. Severe joint space narrowing of shoulder, subchondral sclerosis, subchondral cyst, and osteophyte formation (*arrow*).

Degeneration of articular cartilage is a sign of progression of OA. Plain radiographs cannot detect early chondral damage. Instead, MRI can provide information about size and structural integrity of cartilage. This can be extremely useful in identifying full or partial thickness changes of articular cartilage in OA.[37] MRI can also be used to identify predisposing factors for OA such a meniscal and anterior cruciate ligament injuries (**Fig. 6**).[38,39]

Ultrasound can also assess the synovium for hypertrophy and inflammation. The Rheumatoid Arthritis Clinical Trials Ultrasonography Taskforce defines ultrasound-detected synovial hypertrophy as "abnormal hypoechoic intraarticular tissue that is, nondisplaceable and poorly compressible and which may exhibit Doppler signal."[40] Ultrasound technology offers many advantages, including low cost, lack of ionizing radiation, ability to image structure dynamically, and can be used for interventional procedures. MRI can be used to detect OA in deeper joints such as the hip and shoulder that ultrasound cannot assess.

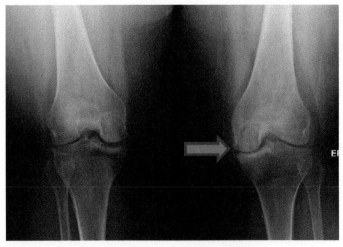

Fig. 5. Severe narrowing of the medial compartment (*arrow*).

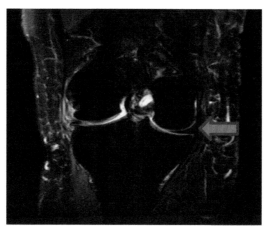

Fig. 6. Medial meniscus. Degenerative oblique tear of the posterior horn (*arrow*).

LABORATORY FINDINGS

Laboratory test results are usually normal in patients with OA, although they may be useful for narrowing the differential diagnoses when the diagnosis is uncertain. C-reactive protein levels and erythrocyte sedimentation rate can be useful to evaluate for systemic inflammatory conditions and autoimmune disorders. A uric acid level may help evaluate for the presence of gout. Clinical guidelines established by the American College of Rheumatology recommend against routine ordering of arthritis panels for patients with joint problems.[41]

DIFFERENTIAL DIAGNOSIS

It is important in the diagnosis and treatment of OA to consider a broad differential. Important alterative diagnoses and differentiating features are identified in **Table 2**. Examination, imaging, laboratory workup, and history can help distinguish these cases when initial evaluation is uncertain.

TREATMENT

There is no current cure for OA. Treatment can be broadly classified into reduction of modifiable risk factors, intraarticular therapy, physical modalities, alternative therapies, and surgical treatments (**Table 3**). There is also emerging evidence for several novel treatments. Early on in the course of OA the treatment is focused on the reduction of pain and stiffness. Later, treatment focuses on maintaining physical functioning.

Nonpharmacologic Treatment

Reduction of modifiable risk factors
Obesity may be the strongest modifiable risk factor. A randomized trial by Messier and colleagues (2011) demonstrated that a 10% reduction in body weight significantly decreased the load in knee joints.[42] Another study demonstrated that the risk of symptomatic knee OA in women decreases by 50% by losing 5 kg of weight.[43] Recent studies also showed structural improvement of cartilage and positive changes in biomarkers of cartilage and bone with weight loss.[44]

Table 2
Differential diagnosis for osteoarthritis

Knee OA	Hip OA	Shoulder OA	Hand OA	Multiple Joint OA
Pes anserine bursitis	Aortoiliac insufficiency	Rotator cuff impingement, tendinopathy, tears	Trigger finger (stenosis flexor tenosynovitis)	Referred pain from another joint or radicular pain
Patellar tendinosis	Referred visceral pain	Labral tear	Ganglion cyst	Osteochondritis dissecans
Patellofemoral pain syndrome	Sacroiliac neuropathy	Adhesvie capsulitis	Dupuytren contracture	Pigmented villonodular synovitis
Prepatellar bursitis	Lateral femoral cutaneous nerve syndrome	Glenohumeral joint or scapular instability	Carpal tunnel syndrome	Avascular necrosis
Semimembranous bursitis	Acetabular labral tear	Biceps tendinopathy	Mallet finger	Gout
Iliotibial band syndrome	Femoroacetabular impingement	Scapulothoracic weakness		Pseudogout
Medial plica syndrome	Greater trochanteric pain syndrome (trochanteric bursitis)	Subscapular bursitis		Septic arthritis
Popliteal cyst, popliteus tendinopathy	Snapping hip	Distal clavicular osteolysis		Traumatic ligamentous or bony injury
Quadriceps tendonosis	Piriformis syndrome	AC joint sprain		Systemic rheumatologic disease: rheumatoid arthritis, psoriatic arthritis, reactive arthritis, hemochromatosis
Popliteal artery aneurysm or entrapment	Osteitis pubis	Sternoclavicular joint subluxation/dislocation		Stress and osteoporotic fracture
Saphenous nerve entrapment	Sacroiliac joint pain			Bone tumors
Hoffa fat pad syndrome				

Data from Refs.[45–49]

Table 3
Treatment options for osteoarthritis with Osteoarthritis Research Society International guidelines (if available)

	Treatment	OARSI Guidelines Recommendation
Reduction in modifiable risk factor	Weight loss	Appropriate
	Exercise	Appropriate: both land and water based, including strengthening
Bracing and physical modalities	Cane	Appropriate for knee-only OA
	Crutches	Uncertain
	Biomechanical interventions	Appropriate
Alternative therapies	T'ai Chi	No recommendation
	Acupuncture	Uncertain
	Balneotherapy/spa	Appropriate with individuals with multiple joint OA Uncertain with knee-only OA
	NMES	Not appropriate
	Self-management and education	Appropriate
	Cognitive behavioral therapy	No recommendation
	TENS	Uncertain in knee-only OA, otherwise inappropriate
	Ultrasound	Uncertain in knee-only OA, otherwise inappropriate
	Laser therapy	No recommendation
	Electromagnetic field therapy	No recommendation
Pharmacologic (oral)	Acetaminophen	Appropriate depending on comorbidities
	Avocado soybean unsaponfiables	Uncertain
	Chondroitin/glucosamine	Uncertain for symptom relief, not appropriate for disease modification
	Diacerein	Uncertain
	Duloxetine	Appropriate with multijoint OA, uncertain in knee-only OA
	NSAIDs	Appropriate in those without significant comorbidities
	Opioids	Uncertain
	Risedronate	Not appropriate
	Rosehip	Uncertain
Pharmacologic (topical)	Capsaicin	Appropriate in knee-only OA
	NSAIDs	Appropriate in knee-only OA, uncertain in multijoint OA
	Tramadol	No recommendation
	Opioids	Uncertain
	Topical NSAIDs	No recommendation
Pharmacologic (intraarticular)	Corticosteroids	Appropriate
	Hyaluronic acid	Uncertain in knee-only OA, not appropriate in multijoint OA

Data from Rannou F, Poiraudeau S, Beaudreuil J. Role of bracing in the management of knee osteoarthritis. Curr Opin Rheumatol 2010;22(2):218–222.

Exercise has also been investigated as a treatment modality for OA. A network meta-analysis of 60 randomized control studies by Uthman and colleagues (2013) found that exercise improved pain and function in individuals with OA. This study also suggested interventions that combined strengthening, flexibility, and aerobic exercise.[45] Aquatic exercise may also be effective.[46]

A Cochrane review of knee arthritis found that exercise led to decreased pain, improved physical function, and mildly improved QOL. The improvement noted was similar to previous studies evaluating nonsteroidal antiinflammatory drugs (NSAIDs).[47]

Most patients would likely benefit from a guided therapy program with a certified physical or occupational therapist before initiating a home exercise program. This allows the patient to have onsite direction and equipment, which may help with program adherence and outcomes. There is limited information to guide specific recommendations in terms of dosing and specific types of exercise.[48,49] Specific therapy techniques that are used include passive stretching, soft tissue mobilization, active range of motion exercises, and progressive muscle strengthening. Specific goals (such as increasing strength, flexibility, and range of motion) are generally progressed with time in a physical therapy program. Specific exercises and techniques for knee OA are outlined in the article by Deyle and colleagues (2005), although similar techniques would be used for other joint locations.

Physical modalities
Although more research is needed, bracing may be effective in treating knee OA. Unloading knee braces may provide some symptomatic relief in medial and lateral knee OA. For patellar OA, sleeves with a peripatellar device or taping may be helpful. For multicompartmental knee braces, neutral knee braces may be effective. Knee sleeves may provide some warmth and relief. Lateral and medial wedge insoles may also be effective in the treatment of OA.[50] For carpometacarpal OA thumb base semirigid and rigid splints can be used to immobilize the joint.

Alternative therapies
Alternative therapies have also been investigated for OA. Study results have been mixed with little definitive support for acupuncture in high-quality studies.[51–55] Despite this, there does not seem to be significant risk associated with knee acupuncture and may prove useful for some patients.[56]

Self-management and education is another potential approach to treat the pain of OA. Self-management is the concept of putting the management of symptoms and consequences of the disease in the hands of the patient. Specific concepts include the following:

- Self-efficacy building
- Self-monitoring
- Goal setting and action planning
- Decision-making
- Problem solving
- Self-tailoring
- Partnership between the views of patients and health professionals

Arthritis self-management programs have been shown to be beneficial and improve pain and disability.[57]

Increased pain with OA has been associated with psychological dysfunction, depression, anxiety, pain catastrophizing, social isolation, and poor coping strategies. Cognitive behavioral therapy, psychotherapy using structured sessions to help individuals identify and modify negative thinking and behaviors, has also been used in the treatment of OA. Studies of CBT have shown mixed outcomes for OA.[58]

Other treatments used such as lasers, transcutaneous electrical nerve stimulation, ultrasound, and electromagnetic field therapy are commonly used but evidence is poor on their effectiveness.[59,60]

Pharmacologic Treatment

NSAIDs and acetaminophen are generally considered first-line therapies in the treatment of OA. NSAIDs are effective for overall pain from OA.[61] There is no strong evidence of benefit of any particular NSAID over another. NSAIDS should be used with caution in those with gastrointestinal disease including selective cox-2 inhibitors or nonselective NSAIDs with the addition of a gastroprotective agent.[62]

Acetaminophen has been found to be effective in the treatment of OA, although modestly. They are also less effective than NSAIDs. Acetaminophen is generally safe and may be preferable when NSAIDs are contraindicated.[61] Topical options such as capsaicin and topical NSAIDs are also available and effective.

Other treatments include serotonin-norepinephrine reuptake inhibitors. Recent evidence has implicated central sensitization as an important factor in pain in OA. There is a theory that limited efficacy by NSAID or acetaminophen occurs because the pain may be central in origin. Both noradrenergic and serotonergic neurons modulate the spinal cord and periaqueductal gray area in the spinal cord. Chapell and colleagues (2011) performed the first randomized controlled trial comparing duloxetine with a placebo. In this trial the patient treated with duloxetine exhibited significant improvements in average pain scores.[63] Another study showed that duloxetine along with an NSAID was more effective than an NSAID alone for pain in OA. This study led to the Food and Drug Administration (FDA) approving duloxetine for the treatment of chronic knee OA.[64]

The use of stronger medications, such as weak opioids and narcotic analgesics, can be considered when other medications have failed or are contraindicated.[65] Physicians should adhere to the new opioid guidelines issued by Center for Disease Control and Prevention in 2016 when treating patients.[66]

Avocado soybean unsaponifiables, glucosamine sulfate, chondroitin sulfate, hyaluronic acid, and diacerein, have also been used by patients for OA with uncertain efficacy.

Intraarticular Treatments

Intraarticular injection of steroids is an option in the treatment of inflammatory flares of OA, although efficacy is limited and short-lived.[62] Viscosupplements such as hyaluronic acid have uncertain effects when used intraarticulately for the treatment of OA in the knee. Although possibly less effective in the short term, they may provide longer-lasting treatment in OA.[67]

Novel Treatments

Recent improvements in the understanding of the pathophysiology of the disease have led to novel treatments.

Strontium ranelate inhibits subchondral bone resorption by regulating the activity of osteoprotegerin, RANK ligand, and matrix metalloproteinases produced by osteoblasts. Strontium may have a direct effect on cartilage; this is supported by the observation that it promotes proteoglycan synthesis, which stimulates cartilage matrix formation in vitro.[68]

Nerve growth factor (NGF) is postulated to modulate signals that control expression of peripheral and central pain substances and sensitizes adjacent nociceptive neurons in response to stimulation. Tanezumab is a highly selective immunoglobulin G2 antibody against NGF. Several studies have shown that in patients with moderate to severe knee OA tanezumab results in greater improvement in knee pain, stiffness, and increase function compared with placebo. However, side effects include osteonecrosis leading to the medication being placed on hold by the FDA.[69]

Regenerative therapy has been one the latest rapidly growing strategies to treat OA. Platelet-rich plasma, which is harvested from a patient's blood with the theory that it will provide important growth factors, has been investigated. A systematic review found that platelet-rich plasma resulted in clinical improvement up to 12 months following injection.[70]

Mesenchymal stem cells (MSCs) are a cell source that can be easily obtained from a variety of tissues such as bone marrow, adipose tissue, and synovium. The stem cells are capable of rapid proliferation, chondro-differentiation and immunosuppression. One study showed mild improvements in pain for 5 years after injection of MSCs into the knee joint.[71,72]

Another area of investigation is the use of radiofrequency ablation in the treatment of knee OA. These procedures thermally lesion sensory nerves, which include the superior lateral and medial and inferior medial genicular nerves of the anterior joint capsule of the knee, in order to decrease pain. To date, results are promising for improvement in pain and reducing disability.[73]

Other novel approaches being investigated include cryotherapy and geniculate arterial embolization.

SURGICAL TREATMENTS

Total joint arthroplasty is the gold standard treatment of patients with severe OA who failed to respond to conservative treatment or pain is severely affecting their QOL. It can provide marked pain relief and functional improvement in patients with severe hip or knee OA. One study found after 12 months surgically treated patients had greater pain relief and improvement in QOL than conservative treatment.[74]

With contemporary techniques, patients are typically allowed to weight bear as tolerated on the affected limb immediately after surgery. Pain control is important and accomplished by a multimodal approach. NSAIDS, analgesics, and narcotics may be used. Patients typical stay in the hospital for 2 or 3 days, although more patients are leaving sooner after surgery.

Prevention of complications early after surgery is critical. Early complications include infections, failed prosthesis, wound dehiscence, and deep vein thrombosis. Pneumonia or atelectasis can be prevented with an incentive spirometer. Thrombotic events are prevented by compression stocking and/or chemical prophylaxis. Active exercises with early and frequent ambulation can also help to prevent thrombosis. Early mobilization on the day of surgery helped to improve outcomes and decrease hospital length of stay.[75]

In order to prevent hip dislocation following total hip arthroplasty (THA), patients are placed on hip precautions. Precautions from a THA done from a direct anterior approach include avoidance of hyperextension, adduction, and external rotation of the hip. For surgery done from a posterior approach the patient should avoid hyperflexion, adduction, and internal rotation of the hip.

There is no clear consensus regarding optimal frequency, duration, or intensity of physical rehabilitation following joint replacement surgery. A well-structured therapy program that includes range of motion, gait training, quadriceps strengthening, and training in activities of daily living is an important component of the rehabilitation process following surgery.

Patients are discharged to home, a skilled nursing facility, or an acute inpatient reha-bilitation hospital. Medicare standards currently allow acute rehabilitation for patients with bilateral total joint arthroplasty, morbid obesity, or age greater than 85 years. Close communication and coordination between hospital facility and the acute reha-bilitation hospital is crucial to prevent complications or readmissions.

THA patients make most functional gains in the first 6 months, and total knee replacement (TKR) can take up to 1 year. Quadriceps strength can be reduced up to 60% after TKR, which can be mitigated by strengthening exercises.[76] These exer-cises will help increase a patient's stair climbing ability, gait speed, and coordination, all of which are crucial for independent living at home. After a TKR, the expected range of motion of the knee is full extension to 90° of flexion. This is the minimum required to be able to perform activities of daily living. Many patients will achieve up to 115% degrees or more. It is not atypical to have swelling and pain up to 1 year after surgery.

SUMMARY

OA is a widespread and devastating condition that leads to pain, diminished QOL, and high health care costs. Because increasing emphasis is being placed on cost-efficient treatment (including increasing use of bundled payments), further work is needed to understand the costs and cost-savings of accurate diagnosis and treatments before surgery and the efficacy of novel treatment options. As we are learning more everyday about the pathogenesis of OA, and that it is not just "wear and tear," it is opening the door to new treatment avenues. Given the multiple pathways involved in the disorder, a multidisciplinary approach to treatment and prevention is likely the future treatment of OA.

DISCLOSURE

The authors have nothing to disclose.

REFERENCES

1. Cisternas Miriam G, Murphy L, Sacks Jeffrey J, et al. Alternative methods for defining osteoarthritis and the impact on estimating prevalence in a US population-based survey. Arthritis Care Res 2016;574–80.
2. James Spencer L, Abate D, Abate Kalkidan H, et al. Global, regional, and na-tional incidence, prevalence, and years lived with disability for 354 Diseases and Injuries for 195 countries and territories, 1990-2017: a systematic analysis for the Global Burden of Disease Study 2017. Lancet 2018;392(10159):1789–858.
3. From the Centers for Disease Control and Prevention. Prevalence and impact of arthritis among women–United States, 1989-1991. JAMA 1995;273(23):1820.
4. Hunter David J, Schofield D, Emily C. The individual and socioeconomic impact of osteoarthritis. Nat Rev Rheumatol 2014;10(7):437–41.
5. Murphy Louise B, Cisternas Miriam G, Pasta David J, et al. Medical expenditures and earnings losses among US adults with arthritis in 2013. Arthritis Care Res 2018;70(6):869–76.
6. Musumeci G, Aiello FC, Szychlinska MA, et al. Osteoarthritis in the XXIst century: risk factors and behaviours that influence disease onset and progression. Int J Mol Sci 2015;16(3):6093–112.
7. Ali M, Batt M. An update on the pathophysiology of osteoarthritis. Ann Phys Re-habil Med 2016;333–9. https://doi.org/10.1016/j.rehab.2016.07.004.

8. Berenbaum F. Osteoarthritis as an inflammatory disease (osteoarthritis is not os-teoarthrosis!). Osteoarthr Cartil 2013;16–21. https://doi.org/10.1016/j.joca.2012.11.012.
9. Yusuf E, Nelissen RG, Ioan-Facsinay A, et al. Association between weight or body mass index and hand osteoarthritis: a systematic review. Ann Rheum Dis 2010;69(4):761–5.
10. Loeser Richard F. Aging and osteoarthritis. Curr Opin Rheumatol 2011;492–6. https://doi.org/10.1097/BOR.0b013e3283494005.
11. Shane Anderson A, Loeser Richard F. Why is osteoarthritis an age-related dis-ease? Best Pract Res Clin Rheumatol 2010;15–26. https://doi.org/10.1016/j.berh.2009.08.006.
12. Murray Christopher JL, Lopez Alan D. The global burden of disease: a compre-hensive assessment of mortality and disability from deceases, injuries and risk factors in 1990 and projected to 2010, vol. 1. Cambridge, MA: Harvard Univ Press; 1996. p. 1–35.
13. Felson David T, Zhang Y, Hannan Marian T, et al. The incidence and natural his-tory of knee osteoarthritis in the elderly, the framingham osteoarthritis study. Arthritis Rheum 1995;38(10):1500–5.
14. Barter MJ, Bui C, Young DA. Epigenetic mechanisms in cartilage and osteoar-thritis: DNA methylation, histone modifications and microRNAs. Osteoarthr Cartil 2012;339–49. https://doi.org/10.1016/j.joca.2011.12.012.
15. Blagojevic M, Jinks C, Jeffery A, et al. Risk factors for onset of osteoarthritis of the knee in older adults: a systematic review and meta-analysis. Osteoarthr Cartil 2010;18(1):24–33.
16. Sellam J, Berenbaum F. Is osteoarthritis a metabolic disease? Joint Bone Spine 2013;568–73. https://doi.org/10.1016/j.jbspin.2013.09.007.
17. Hunter DJ, March L, Sambrook PN. Knee osteoarthritis: the influence of environ-mental factors. Clin Exp Rheumatol 2002;20(1):93–100.
18. Prieto-Alhambra D, Judge A, Javaid MK, et al. Incidence and risk factors for clin-ically diagnosed knee, hip and hand osteoarthritis: Influences of age, gender and osteoarthritis affecting other joints. Ann Rheum Dis 2014;73(9):1659–64.
19. Brown TD, Johnston Richard C, Saltzman Charles L, et al. Posttraumatic osteoar-thritis: a first estimate of incidence, prevalence, and burden of disease. J Orthop Trauma 2006;20:739–44.
20. Thomas Abbey C, Hubbard-Turner T, Wikstrom Erik A, et al. Epidemiology of posttraumatic osteoarthritis. J Athl Train 2016;52(6):491–6.
21. Coggon D, Croft P, Samantha K, et al. Occupational physical activities and oste-oarthritis of the knee. Arthritis Rheum 2000;43(7):1443–9.
22. Allen Kelli D, Chen JC, Callahan Leigh F, et al. Associations of occupational tasks with knee and hip osteoarthritis: The Johnston County Osteoarthritis Project. J Rheumatol 2010;37(4):842–50.
23. Sandmark H, Hogstedt C, Vingård E. Primary osteoarthrosis of the knee in men and women as a result of lifelong physical load from work. Scand J Work Environ Health 2000;26(1):20–5.
24. Cameron Kenneth L, Hsiao Mark S, Owens Brett D, et al. Incidence of physician-diagnosed osteoarthritis among active duty United States military service mem-bers. Arthritis Rheum 2011;63(10):2974–82.
25. Kujala Urho M, Kettunen J, Paananen H, et al. Knee osteoarthritis in former run-ners, soccer players, weight lifters, and shooters. Arthritis Rheum 1995;38(4):539–46.

26. Woolf Anthony D, Bruce P. Burden of major musculoskeletal conditions. Bull World Health Organ 2003;646–56.
27. Zhang Y, Jordan Joanne M. Epidemiology of osteoarthritis. Clinics in geriatric medicine, vol. 26. NIH Public Access; 2010. p. 355–69.
28. Allen Kelli D, Golightly Yvonne M. Epidemiology of osteoarthritis: state of the evidence. Curr Opin Rheumatol 2015;276–83. https://doi.org/10.1097/BOR.0000000000000161.
29. Hawker GA, Stewart L, French MR, et al. Understanding the pain experience in hip and knee osteoarthritis - an OARSI/OMERACT initiative. Osteoarthr Cartil 2008;16(4):415–22.
30. Neogi T. The epidemiology and impact of pain in osteoarthritis. Osteoarthr Cartil 2013;21(9):1145–53.
31. Altman R, Alarcón G, Appelrouth D, et al. The American College of Rheumatology criteria for the classification and reporting of osteoarthritis of the hip. Arthritis Rheum 1991;34(5):505–14.
32. Bruno F, Pascal H, Rozenberg S, et al. Impact of osteoarthritis: results of a nationwide survey of 10 000 patients consulting for OA. Rev Du Rhum 2005;72(5 SPEC. ISS.):404–10.
33. Salaffi F, Carotti M, Stancati A, et al. Health-related quality of life in older adults with symptomatic hip and knee osteoarthritis: a comparison with matched healthy controls. Aging Clin Exp Res 2005;17(4):255–63.
34. Goodman S. Osteoarthritis. In: Yee AMF, Paget SA, editors. Expert guide to rheumatology. Philadelphia: American College of Physicians; 2005. p. 269–83.
35. Kellgren JH, Lawrence JS. Radiological assessment of osteo-arthrosis. Ann Rheum Dis 1957;16(4):494–502.
36. Kohn Mark D, Sassoon Adam A, Fernando Navin D. Classifications in brief: Kellgren-Lawrence classification of osteoarthritis. Clin Orthop Relat Res 2016; 474(8):1886–93.
37. Potter HG, Linklater JM, Allen AA, et al. Magnetic resonance imaging of articular cartilage in the knee. An evaluation with use of fast-spin-echo imaging. J Bone Joint Surg Am 1998;80(9):1276–84.
38. Song Y, Greve JM, Carter DR, et al. Meniscectomy alters the dynamic deformational behavior and cumulative strain of tibial articular cartilage in knee joints subjected to cyclic loads. Osteoarthr Cartil 2008;16(12):1545–54.
39. Lohmander LS, Englund PM, Dahl LL, et al. The long-term consequence of anterior cruciate ligament and meniscus injuries: osteoarthritis. Am J Sports Med 2007;1756–69. https://doi.org/10.1177/0363546507307396.
40. Wakefield Richard J, Balint Peter V, Szkudlarek M, et al. Musculoskeletal ultrasound including definitions for ultrasonographic pathology. J Rheumatol 2005; 32:2485–7.
41. Shmerling Robert H, Fuchs Howard A, Lorish Christopher D, et al. Guidelines for the initial evaluation of the adult patient with acute musculoskeletal symptoms. Arthritis Rheum 1996;1–8. https://doi.org/10.1002/art.1780390102.
42. Messier SP, Legault C, Loeser RF, et al. Does high weight loss in older adults with knee osteoarthritis affect bone-on-bone joint loads and muscle forces during walking? Osteoarthr Cartil 2011;19(3):272–80.
43. Pai YC, Rymer WZ, Chang Rowland W, et al. Effect of age and osteoarthritis on knee proprioception. Arthritis Rheum 1997;40(12):2260–5.
44. Anandacoomarasamy A, Leibman S, Smith G, et al. Weight loss in obese people has structure-modifying effects on medial but not on lateral knee articular cartilage. Ann Rheum Dis 2012;71(1):26–32.

45. Uthman OA, van der Windt DA, Jordan JL, et al. Exercise for lower limb osteoarthritis: systematic review incorporating trial sequential analysis and network meta-analysis. BMJ 2013;347(sep20 1):f5555.
46. Hinman Rana S, Heywood Sophie E, Day Anthony R. Aquatic physical therapy for hip and knee osteoarthritis: results of a single-blind randomized controlled trial. Phys Ther 2007;87(1):32–43.
47. Fransen M, Mcconnell S, Harmer Alison R, et al. Exercise for osteoarthritis of the knee. Cochrane Database Syst Rev 2015:CD004376. https://doi.org/10.1002/14651858.CD004376.pub3.
48. Bhatia D, Bejarano T, Novo M. Current interventions in the management of knee osteoarthritis. J Pharm Bioallied Sci 2013;5(1):30.
49. Deyle Gail D, Allison Stephen C, Matekel Robert L, et al. Physical therapy treatment effectiveness for osteoarthritis of the knee: a randomized comparison of supervised clinical exercise and manual therapy procedures versus a home exercise program. Phys Ther 2005;85(12):1301–17.
50. Rannou F, Poiraudeau S, Beaudreuil J. Role of bracing in the management of knee osteoarthritis. Curr Opin Rheumatol 2010;218–22. https://doi.org/10.1097/BOR.0b013e32833619c4.
51. Manheimer Eric, Cheng Ke, Wieland LS, et al. Acupuncture for hip osteoarthritis. Cochrane Database Syst Rev 2018. https://doi.org/10.1002/14651858.CD013010.
52. Manheimer E, Cheng K, Linde K, et al. Acupuncture for peripheral joint osteoarthritis. Cochrane Database Syst Rev 2010. https://doi.org/10.1002/14651858.CD001977.pub2.
53. Kwon YD, Pittler Max H, Ernst E. Acupuncture for peripheral joint osteoarthritis. Rheumatology 2006;1331–7. https://doi.org/10.1093/rheumatology/kel207.
54. Ezzo J, Hadhazy V, Birch S, et al. Acupuncture for osteoarthritis of the knee: a systematic review. Arthritis Rheum 2001;44(4):819–25.
55. Manyanga T, Froese M, Zarychanski R, et al. Pain management with acupuncture in osteoarthritis: a systematic review and meta-analysis. BMC Complement Altern Med 2014;14(1):312.
56. Zhang Q, Yue J, Golianu B, et al. Updated systematic review and meta-analysis of acupuncture for chronic knee pain. Acupunct Med 2017;392–403. https://doi.org/10.1136/acupmed-2016-011306.
57. Du S, Yuan C, Xiao X, et al. Self-management programs for chronic musculoskeletal pain conditions: a systematic review and meta-analysis. Patient Educ Couns 2011;e299–310. https://doi.org/10.1016/j.pec.2011.02.021.
58. Helminen EE, Sinikallio Sanna H, Valjakka Anna L, et al. Effectiveness of a cognitive-behavioural group intervention for knee osteoarthritis pain: a randomized controlled trial. Clin Rehabil 2015;29(9):868–81.
59. Welch V, Brosseau L, Peterson J, et al. Therapeutic ultrasound for osteoarthritis of the knee. In: Welch V, editor. Cochrane database of systematic reviews. Chichester (United Kingdom): John Wiley & Sons, Ltd; 2001:CD003132.
60. Rutjes Anne WS, Nüesch E, Sterchi R, et al. Therapeutic ultrasound for osteoarthritis of the knee or hip. Cochrane Database Syst Rev 2010;(1):CD003132.
61. Towheed T, Maxwell L, Judd M, et al. Acetaminophen for osteoarthritis. Cochrane Database Syst Rev 2006;(1):CD004257.
62. Bennell Kim L, Hunter David J, Hinman Rana S. Management of osteoarthritis of the knee. BMJ 2012;345:e4934.
63. Chappell Amy S, Desaiah D, Liu-Seifert H, et al. A double-blind, randomized, placebo-controlled study of the efficacy and safety of duloxetine for the treatment of chronic pain due to osteoarthritis of the knee. Pain Pract 2011;11(1):33–41.

64. Brown Jacques P, Boulay Luc J. Clinical experience with duloxetine in the management of chronic musculoskeletal pain. A focus on osteoarthritis of the knee. Ther Adv Musculoskelet Dis 2013;291–304. https://doi.org/10.1177/1759720X13508508.
65. Zhang W, Moskowitz RW, Nuki G, et al. OARSI recommendations for the management of hip and knee osteoarthritis, Part II: OARSI evidence-based, expert consensus guidelines. Osteoarthr Cartil 2008;16(2):137–62.
66. Dowell D, Haegerich Tamara M, Chou R. CDC guideline for prescribing opioids for chronic pain-United States, 2016. JAMA 2016;315(15):1624–45.
67. Yu Shirley P, Hunter David J. Managing osteoarthritis. Aust Prescr 2015;38(4):115–9.
68. Reginster Jean Y, Badurski J, Bellamy N, et al. Efficacy and safety of strontium ranelate in the treatment of knee osteoarthritis: results of a double-blind, randomised placebo-controlled trial. Ann Rheum Dis 2013;72(2):179–86.
69. Brown Mark T, Murphy Frederick T, Radin David M, et al. Tanezumab reduces osteoarthritic hip pain: results of a randomized, double-blind, placebo-controlled phase III trial. Arthritis Rheum 2013;65(7):1795–803.
70. Meheux CJ, McCulloch PC, Lintner DM, et al. Efficacy of intra-articular platelet-rich plasma injections in knee osteoarthritis: a systematic review. Arthroscopy 2016;32(3):495–505.
71. Koh YG, Choi YJ. Infrapatellar fat pad-derived mesenchymal stem cell therapy for knee osteoarthritis. Knee 2012;19(6):902–7.
72. Wu Y, Goh EL, Wang D, et al. Novel treatments for osteoarthritis: an update. Open Access Rheumatol 2018;135–40. https://doi.org/10.2147/OARRR.S176666.
73. Goldman DT, Piechowiak R, Nissman D, et al. Current concepts and future directions of minimally invasive treatment for knee pain. Curr Rheumatol Rep 2018;54. https://doi.org/10.1007/s11926-018-0765-x.
74. Skou Søren T, Roos Ewa M, Laursen Mogens B, et al. A randomized, controlled trial of total knee replacement. N Engl J Med 2015;373(17):1597–606.
75. Chen Antonia F, Stewart Melissa K, Heyl Alma E, et al. Effect of immediate postoperative physical therapy on length of stay for total joint arthroplasty patients. J Arthroplasty 2012;27(6):851–6.
76. Bade Michael J, Stevens-Lapsley Jennifer E. Restoration of physical function in patients following total knee arthroplasty: an update on rehabilitation practices. Curr Opin Rheumatol 2012;208–14. https://doi.org/10.1097/BOR.0b013e32834ff26d.

Common Injuries of the Weekend Athlete

Mark I. Ellen, MD[a],*, Christina Lin, MD[b,1]

KEYWORDS

- Athletic injuries • Weekend warrior weekend athlete • Diagnosis • Treatment

KEY POINTS

- Unlike previous generations, many patients remain in a wide variety of athletic activities later into their lives, some well beyond retirement.
- As the population ages and their activities continue, they are subject to injury of various forms, affecting all aspects of their bodies.
- Injuries to those involved with athletic endeavors or others with limited exposures are relatively common and seen extensively by practitioners with office-based practices.
- Early and accurate diagnosis coupled with relatively simple but timely treatment can make all the difference in returning these weekend warriors to their favorite avocational activities.

INTRODUCTION

Weekend athletes can be defined as individuals who engage in physically demanding recreational sporting activities typically on the weekends despite minimal physical activity during the work week.[1] These are individuals who jump into a high-intensity workout regimen or a new sport without the proper preparation, leading to an increased risk of injury. Weekend athletes lack the time and resources that are normally allocated to elite athletes. Although elite athletes continuously strive to meet a perfect standard both mentally and physically, weekend athletes perform solely for pleasure. These limitations affect their ability to warm up adequately, maintain proper form, avoid fatigue, and in some instances have suitable fitting or working equipment. All of these issues can singly or in combination lead to injury.

Because these weekend athletes often are seen first in a primary care setting with their musculoskeletal injuries and complaints, primary care providers must be able to diagnose and manage many common upper and lower extremity injuries and know when to refer severe injuries to specialists. The following types of injuries are typical

[a] 4230 Marden Way, Birmingham, AL 35242, USA; [b] Department of Physical Medicine and Rehabilitation, Johns Hopkins School of Medicine, Baltimore, MD, USA
[1] Present address: 103 South Gay Street, Apartment 810, Baltimore, MD 21202.
* Corresponding author.
E-mail address: miemd@mac.com

Med Clin N Am 104 (2020) 313–325
https://doi.org/10.1016/j.mcna.2019.10.010
0025-7125/20/© 2019 Elsevier Inc. All rights reserved.

medical.theclinics.com

of what are seen in the senior author's sports medicine practice over the past 3 decades, and the treatment protocols are used to help these individuals return to athletics and minimize future risk of injury.

ACROMIOCLAVICULAR JOINT INJURIES

The shoulder represents a fair amount of injuries that present to the primary care provider. Direct or indirect trauma, overuse, breakdown in form, and improper use of equipment all can lead to pain, dysfunction, and injury to the shoulder girdle. Acromioclavicular (AC) joint injuries are among the most common shoulder injuries in athletes and account for 40% to 50% of shoulder injuries in contact sports.[2] Most injuries occur from a direct contact force to the acromion, with the arm typically adducted, displacing the acromion downward.[3] In some circumstances, an upward force placed through an outstretched hand and arm while falling or a strong downward pull about the upper extremity may cause disruption to the AC joint indirectly.

The Rockwood classification system is used to define AC joint injuries based on the severity of damage to the ligaments about the joint.[4] Type 1 injuries are the mildest in nature. They result in a sprain of the AC joint, leaving the AC ligament and coracoclavicular (CC) ligament intact and the deltoid and trapezius muscular attachments intact. On examination, there is tenderness over the AC joint and full range of motion (ROM) of the shoulder with mild pain. They have a normal appearance on plain Zanca view (bilateral shoulders and same cassette) radiographs. Treatment consists of rest of the area with a sling for 24 hours to 48 hours, local ice, nonsteroidal anti-inflammatory drugs (NSAIDS), and progressive ROM, and rotator cuff strengthening with physical therapy typically is recommended. Patients can return to sports when asymptomatic and have full ROM.

Type 2 injuries occur when the AC ligament tears, the CC ligament is sprained but intact, and the deltoid and trapezius remain attached. Examination reveals tenderness of the AC joint and CC interval with very mild displacement of the AC joint that may be observed on thinner patients. Shoulder ROM tends to be painful, especially with abduction. Radiographs reveal mild elevation of the distal clavicle and slightly increased CC interval. Treatment remains nonoperative and consists of relative rest of the area, a sling for 2 days to 3 days and early gentle ROM followed by a strengthening program for the rotator cuff and shoulder girdle.[5] Chronic type 2 injuries may lead to persistent symptoms, and distal clavicle resection for these cases may be an option.[6]

Type 3 injuries occur when there is complete disruption of the AC and CC ligaments, and the deltoid and trapezius typically are partially detached. Examination reveals tenderness of the AC joint with displacement, distal clavicle, and CC interval with painful ROM in all planes. There is gross motion at the AC joint. Radiographs show the CC interval is increased versus the opposite shoulder by 25% to 100%.[3] Treatment is patient-specific and dependent on a patient's physical requirements.[7] Patients with minimal overhead lifting or throwing requirements may do well nonoperatively with either a sling or figure-8 shoulder harness. This typically allows for earlier return to athletics due to overall shorter treatment period and greater patient comfort. The deformity usually remains, however, and symptoms return as the patient fatigues with increased workloads. More aggressive conservative treatment includes sling with harness device for 6 weeks, holding the distal clavicle depressed and the shoulder elevated. This helps ameliorate the cosmetic deformity. Treatment time, however, is relatively longer. There may be skin complications from the pressure induced by the harness.

Type 4 injuries occur with complete disruption of the AC joint and the clavicle is displaced posteriorly into the trapezius. The CC ligaments typically are disrupted, but both deltoid and trapezius muscles are detached. Patients typically report greater pain than those with type 3 injuries. Examination reveals posterior displacement of the clavicle. Radiographs reveal the extent of posterior displacement of the clavicle, best seen on axillary view. Treatment typically is surgical with open reduction and stabilization techniques in acute cases, and chronic injuries also may require distal clavicle resection with or without a CC reconstruction.[8]

Type 5 injuries are similar to type 3 injuries but represent greater displacement of the AC joint, with the CC interval increased to 100% to 300% versus the opposite shoulder on radiograph.[9] The deltoid and the trapezius muscles are detached as well. Clinically, the patient experiences a greater amount of pain. When compared with type 3 injuries, examination shows larger step-off at the AC joint, greater tenting of the skin over the distal clavicle, and greater shoulder droop appearance. For treatment, most young and athletic patients choose to undergo a surgery to attain near normal anatomy.[10] Older patients with less physical demands may elect nonoperative management with sling and physical therapy aimed at strengthening the rotator cuff, scapular stabilizers, and shoulder girdle. Symptomatic treatment with short-term utilization of ice and NSAIDS.

Type 6 injuries occur when not only are there the same acquired injuries as in type 5 but also the distal clavicle becomes fixed beneath the coracoid or acromion. Radiograph shows a reversal in the CC interval, and clinically they may be associated with more complex neurovascular issues. Therefore, careful assessment of the distal vasculature and nerves is required on examination. Patients appear with flattening of the shoulder contour and extreme pain with limited shoulder ROM. Treatment typically is surgical, requiring anatomic reduction with stabilization of the shoulder joint. More chronic symptoms may require distal clavicle resection with reconstruction of the CC ligaments.[11]

ROTATOR CUFF INJURIES

Rotator cuff injuries commonly are seen in both weekend and elite athletes. Overuse injuries to the shoulder usually are associated with repetitive activities, including overhead heavy lifting, throwing in baseball, and serving in tennis or volleyball but also may include contact sports, such as football. The prevalence of rotator cuff injury due to degenerative changes also increases with age.[12]

Rotator cuff pain is usually referred to the area of the middle deltoid near its insertion, pain anteriorly, superior;y or posteriorly is typically referred pain from a secondary process, such as bicipital tendinopathy and scapular instability. Evaluation for rotator cuff injury consists of history; specific shoulder examination tests that evaluate passive and active ROMs of the shoulder girdle in multiple planes, including external and internal rotation; impingement signs; individual muscle strength testing; scapular kinematics observation; and neurologic testing as needed.[13] Positive findings include weakness elicited by manual muscle testing of the rotator cuff and shoulder girdle musculature, inability to contract the rotator cuff muscles fully, and lack of full ROM with pain.

Radiographs often appear normal in the acute setting of rotator cuff injury. Superior displacement of the humeral head to the border of the undersurface of the acromion, sclerosis of the undersurface of the acromion or footplate of the supraspinatus tendon, cystic changes within the humeral head, and subacromial spurring may be seen with larger or more chronic injuries.[14] Plain radiographs are helpful when performed with true anteroposterior, axillary, and supraspinatus outlet views, as is typical of the senior author's practice.[15]

Treatment consists of relative rest of the area, local icing, and an oral NSAID for 5 days to 7 days. A corticosteroid injection can be offered if a patient is in great pain, unable to bear weight on the affected extremity, or awakened more than a few times at night per week.[16] Physical therapy is beneficial to help diminish inflammation, improve ROM of the glenohumeral joint, and strengthen the rotator cuff muscles. The senior author recommends the exercises be performed isotonically with light free weights or resistance bands and doing 3 sets of 8 repetitions to 12 repetitions per exercise twice per week. Patients should start with a limited number of exercises first to gain an excellent understanding of form before progressing 2 to 3 additional exercises every 2 weeks to 3 weeks.

If no improvement after a few weeks of conservative management, further radiologic work-up may be helpful. Ultrasonography has made tremendous advances in the past 2 decades to help evaluate the integrity of the rotator cuff tendons. This remains dependent, however, on the skill of the operator.[17] Magnetic resonance imaging (MRI) continues to represent the gold standard for imaging.[18] With each decade, however, over age 40, the MRI becomes less specific because chronic changes within the shoulder joints lead to signal changes that may be confused with acute injury. In the mature patient, the MRI findings must be correlated with the physical examination and patient complaints. If there continues to be no improvement after 3 months to 6 months of conservative management, surgical consultation is recommended. Traumatic rotator cuff injuries usually are treated surgically.[19] Chronic full-thickness tears are treated surgically if the patient is symptomatic. There is weak evidence that surgical repair of asymptomatic partial or full-thickness rotator cuff tears offers better outcomes than nonsurgical management.[20]

ELBOW EPICONDYLITIS INJURIES

Both golf and tennis have been described as lifetime sports because they can be played to the last day.[21] Not everyone, however, can play as regularly as they wish, have correct form, or have the appropriate equipment. Elbow epicondylitis has been reported to be more dominant in the fourth and fifth decades, with a nearly equal male-to-female ratio.[22] Epicondylitis is a broad term given to injuries in the elbow region. It actually is a misnomer because the epicondyle is not inflamed or involved, and no inflammatory cells have been noted on histology.[23,24] Rather it is thought that mechanical overload at the elbow leads to fibrodysplasia at the bone-tendon interface as the etiology.

Elbow epicondylitis is a clinical diagnosis.[25] On physical examination for lateral epicondylitis, or tennis elbow, there is lateral elbow tenderness, pain worse with wrist extension, and finger extension against resistance, whereas for medial epicondylitis, or golfer's elbow, there is medial elbow tenderness and pain worse with wrist flexion against extension. For treatment, the authors have found that splinting the wrist with a simple resting wrist splint in neutral position during the day limits the common flexor or extensor muscles active actions. In combination with local icing and stretching, most of a patient's pain can be eliminated. Formal physical therapy with wrist splinting has been found to be a beneficial adjunct in the care of epicondylitis about the elbow.[26]

Injections are still beneficial in those patients with pain at night, intractable pain, failure of other methods, or a limited time horizon, such as an important game in which they wish to participate in fully. The standard of choice for injections of elbow epicondylitis remains corticosteroid. Plasma-rich plasma (PRP) injection has been shown effective as well, but for many it remains out of reach due to cost.[27]

ULNAR COLLATERAL LIGAMENT INJURIES OF THE THUMB

Winter sports are enjoyed by a vast percentage of the population and also are considered lifelong sports. Injuries to the ulnar collateral ligament (UCL) of the thumb are common in skiing, typically occurring when the thumb is caught within a constrained space, such as the strap of a ski pole causing a forced abduction of the thumb, resulting in a tear of the UCL either within its substance or from its bony insertion.[28] The UCL comprises the proper collateral ligament, which resists valgus forces during thumb flexion, and the accessory collateral ligament, which resists valgus forces during thumb extension.

Patients complain of pain over the ulnar portion of the base at the metacarpal phalangeal joint. On examination, inspection reveals swelling of the area and palpation confirms tenderness and may reveal the palpable mass of the retracted tendon and/or the bony avulsion seen with some injuries. Comparing the affected side with the non-injured side, instability is noted with the application of stress to the metacarpophalangeal (MCP) joint with the thumb flexed to 30°. This is consistent with an injury to the proper ligament. Instability with valgus stress while the thumb is in neutral position is typical of an injury to both the accessory and common ligaments and may incorporate injury to the volar plate.[29] Plain radiographs of posteroanterior and oblique and lateral views of the thumb should be obtained to evaluate for volar plate and condylar occult fractures, rotation of the proximal phalanx, or volar subluxation of the proximal phalanx, indicating further capsular damage. Further imaging, such as ultrasound and MRI, can be useful adjunct modalities but usually are not necessary.

Nonoperative treatment is immobilization of the joint for those with partial ruptures of the UCL injuries and less than 20° of instability on examination. A thumb spica splint in these patients may be utilized with good results.[30] Some patients with more demanding vocations or physical endeavors or those who may not be compliant may be best placed in a short arm thumb spica cast to protect the UCL. Immobilization for 6 weeks to 8 weeks is recommended. After completion with thumb immobilization, a short course of outpatient occupational therapy is helpful in order to return to full activity.

A Stener lesion is a complete tear of the UCL from the proximal thumb at the level of the MCP joint. These injuries require surgical fixation to allow for proper healing.[31] After UCL surgical repair, there is postoperative immobilization of the ligament with a plaster cast or thermoplastic splint for 4 weeks to 8 weeks. The plaster cast, however, can be more uncomfortable and lead to stiffness of the thumb. One study showed that a spica splint allowed for flexion and extension of the MCP joint, and it led to faster and better functional recovery compared with the group with the plaster cast. Another study, however, showed the functional results to be the same.[32,33] After 6 weeks of immobilization, gentle ROM of the hand with physical therapy can be started. It can take approximately 3 months for the pain to subside and ROM to completely return.[34] For patients with a chronic UCL injury, surgery is generally indicated because chronic instability can result in chronic pain and development of osteoarthritis.[35]

ILIOTIBIAL BAND SYNDROME

Weekend athletes have limited time to work out and enjoy their chosen athletic endeavors. Their workout intensity, frequency, and length can be markedly varied within short durations of time. Appropriate warm-up and stretching may not happen due to time constraints of work or a busy schedule. This can lead to many people choosing to schedule more intense or longer duration workouts on their days off. These may include longer bicycle rides, runs, hikes, or simple walks. Increased risk factors for sport injuries include age-related changes to collagen tissue that decrease flexibility, prior injury to that same area, improper warm-up, fatigue, muscles that have high proportion of type II fast twitch fibers, and crossing of multiple joints.[36] Muscles or fibrous tissues that cross 2 joints are placed at a higher risk because of lengthening loads at both joints at the same time and mixed demands during the activity.[37]

One common example is the iliotibial (IT) band, which crosses both the hip and knee joints laterally. It originates from the tensor fascia lata and inserts distally on the Gerdy tubercle at the anterolateral tibia. If not appropriately stretched, it may not be flexible enough to withstand increased tensile loads associated with increased time or intensity of athletic activity and may lead to shortening of individual fiber length. This fiber shortening is seen on examination as tightness of the IT band with Ober test and pain with palpation either over the greater trochanteric bursa or insertion site of Gerdy tubercle.[38] The trochanteric bursa can become irritated as the IT band slides repeatedly over the bursa, and, as the IT band tightens, there is more pressure placed on the bursa.[39] Pain is noted laterally about the hip and it may radiate down the leg to the level of the knee.

Treatment is conservative management of local icing, oral NSAIDs, and most importantly, stretching of the IT band frequently throughout the day as well as prior to, during, and after activity. Some patients need more guidance and may need a short course of outpatient physical therapy for a flexibility program or modalities, such as electric stimulation, cross-friction massage, and dry needling, in order to respond. Decreasing time of the offending activity to less than when symptoms first began or when pain becomes noticeably increased is also recommended. Once symptoms seem under control, patients may increase the length of time of activity by 5% to 10% every 3 days to 4 days as tolerated. If symptomatic, they should return to prior asymptomatic level of activity and hold there for a week or 2 before slowly increasing activity again.

Corticosteroid injections with or without ultrasonic guidance have been found beneficial in the short term for those with recurrent symptoms or for those who must perform an important activity.[40] PRP, mesenchymal stems cells, and other injectables have not been shown superior to a corticosteroid injection.[41]

PATELLAR TENDINITIS

Patellar tendinitis is believed to be caused by overuse, and it has been related to jumping sports, such as volleyball and basketball. It is perhaps a misnomer with regard to inflammation of the tendon. Studies have revealed no evidence of a cellular inflammatory response.[42] Rather, histologic changes were more consistent with a degenerative process of the collagen fibers with interrupted and disorganized collagen bundles. This has led many to now describe this entity as a tendinosis rather than a tendinitis. There are other studies, however, that note the increase of cytokines, prostaglandins, and other mediators of inflammation in patellar tendinitis seen on biopsies and refute the theory of it being a pure overload injury to the patellar tendon.[43,44]

Various internal and external factors have been studied in order to help determine the cause of patellar tendinitis. The external roles of length of time played and firmer surfaces seem to have the largest role in development of the injury, and the main intrinsic factor seems to be the flexibility of the quadriceps and hamstrings.[45]

Patients report recent increase or change of activity level, lack of warm-up or stretching, prolonged level of activity, and more rarely direct trauma to the knee. Clinically, patients describe sharp knee pain with flexion weight-bearing activities, especially with kneeling, running, or stair climbing. They also may note a sense of local fullness or numbness of the knee. On examination, there is point tenderness just infe-rior to the patella.

Treatment is nonoperative except in the most recalcitrant cases, where fibroblastic changes are noted on MRI and all nonoperative treatments have failed.[46] Treatment should focus on decreasing the load on the patellar tendon by decreasing activity level. The authors have found that most patients do not require a complete shutdown of athletic endeavors. They should expect an initial pain, which should subside after some time. The pain typically returns as the lower extremity musculature fatigues and the load on the patellar tendon increases. Therefore, patients should stop the ac-tivity prior to this occurring. A lower extremity flexibility program, with focus on quad-riceps and hamstring stretching, should be started and performed several times throughout the day, including before and after activity. When combined with gentle icing, many patients had marked decrease in symptoms. Some patients may require an oral NSAID for pain relief, but the authors have not seen this in most patients. Some patients may need further reassurance and may benefit from a course of outpatient physical therapy to help with flexibility and add modalities, such as electric stimulation, phonophoresis, and cross-friction massage.

Corticosteroid injections are known for weakening tendons when directly injected.[46] They should be performed only on the most limited basis with the knowledge that the tendon already has disruptions at the cellular level; therefore, it is not a normal tough bundle of collagen fibers. PRP injections have shown some benefit in patellar tendino-pathies and would be considered much more favorably than corticosteroid injec-tions.[47] After undergoing PRP injection, patients should be shut down for several weeks in order for the growth factors and other mediators of healing to have the chance to work. Extracorporeal shock wave therapy is another treatment option that has shown some benefit, but it does carry an increased risk of full-thickness tendon tear.[48] It can be considered in patients who have failed all other conservative managements.

MENISCAL TEARS

The menisci are made up of fibrocartilage arranged in a cross-linked pattern. They tend to be fairly stable against compressive and straight sheer loads, but they are frag-ile when torque and compressive loads are applied.[49] The collagen substrate also loses elasticity as part of the normal aging process and leads to easier failure of the meniscus. Meniscus injuries typically occur with a twisting force applied to the knee with or without weight bearing. There usually is no other contact force involved.

Knee pain and associated swelling can occur immediately or, more typically, several hours after the inciting event. On physical examination, knee ROM is limited, more so in flexion. The McMurray test may be positive.[50] The knee locking, inability to fully straighten knee, swelling, and joint line tenderness are other findings that patients may report or be seen on examination.[51] The knee locks due to part of the torn meniscus folds into the notch of the femur, and it occupies the space required for further ROM. When locked, gentle traction and rotation about the knee may allow the trapped fragment to slide back and scar down into place. In those patients whose knee remains fixed, an immediate referral to an orthopedic surgeon is indicated for surgical arthroscopy of the knee.

Treatment of meniscal tears is stepwise and consists of relative rest of the knee, local icing, oral NSAID, and then physical therapy. Formal physical therapy consists of modalities to the vastus medialis obliques muscle, gentle and careful ROM of knee, and a protected and careful progressive strengthening regimen of the quadriceps, hamstrings, and calf musculature. Corticosteroid or PRP injections can be considered to reduce local synovitis and pain. Recent studies have shown that PRP injections in open or arthroscopic meniscus repairs resulted in some improvement with meniscus healing and functional outcomes.[52] Bracing can help in a variety of ways. The authors prefer to utilize off the shelf hinged knee braces with free ROM. This allows full weight bearing on an extended knee with some of the load forces being borne by the hinges of the brace for increased patient comfort.

Nonoperative care remains the current standard of care for those with pain and no mechanical symptoms.[53] For patients without findings of knee osteoarthritis and who have true mechanical symptoms of locking, palpable click at the joint line, recurrent swelling or definitive decrease in ROM, however, ordering an MRI or surgical referral after failure of a conservative management is reasonable.[46]

KNEE LIGAMENT INJURIES

The most common type of knee injuries is ligament sprains. The medial collateral ligament (MCL) is the most common and the anterior cruciate ligament (ACL) is the second most commonly sprained.[54] The MCL and ACL are at risk from both contact and noncontact sports. Sudden stopping, cutting to the side, or missing a step while descending steps may injure either of these 2 ligaments. Common sport activities that ligament injuries are seen in are skiing, basketball, football, hockey, and soccer.

On examination of the knee for MCL or ACL injury, there may be swelling, tenderness of the ligament, lack of a firm end point with valgus stressing of the MCL, or positive Lachman test for the ACL. Ultrasound can be used to evaluate the integrity of the collateral ligaments or MRI can be ordered if considering surgical repair.[55] Treatment of ACL injuries is based on a patient's physical requirements. Younger more active patients benefit from elective surgical reconstruction of the ligament. For older patients, however, because the ACL has a limited blood supply that decreases with age, injury to the ACL tends to be complete and permanent.

MCL injuries may be a partial or complete tear. MCL injuries have a better prognosis compared with ACL injuries. The MCL can heal back into place independently. Protective knee bracing with a hinged knee brace for 4 weeks to 6 weeks while limiting knee flexion initially to less than 45° and gradually increasing ROM during the rehabilitative phase protects the ligament from undue traction while allowing some stress to help healing.

Nonoperative management for ACL injuries of oral NSAIDs, local ice, a hinged knee brace, and weight bearing with ambulation as tolerated are initiated immediately. Achieving full extension and increasing hamstring and calf strength are goals of rehabilitation, which should be started as soon as possible.[56] For those who choose nonoperative management, long-term bracing of the knee for athletics or high-level activity is reasonable.[57] Patients with knee injuries should remember that they would be best served on a long-term strengthening program for their lower extremities.

MUSCLE STRAINS

Muscle strains of the calf can occur due to eccentric overload when the knee is extended and the foot is dorsiflexed. The gastrocnemius muscle and its tendons cross 3 joints: the knee, ankle, and subtalar. Eccentric load places the gastrocnemius muscle bellies at risk for load failure. Tearing or straining of the calf muscle fibers occurs when the lower extremity is eccentrically loaded, and the forces generated by either repetitive load, such as running a hilly course, or a quick and powerful change in direction, such as in softball or tennis. It is more common to injure the medial head than the lateral head of the gastrocnemius muscle.[58]

With age, risk of calf injury also increases because the collagen becomes less elastic, and its ability to withstand eccentric load diminishes.[59] Another common reason for calf injury is that most weekend athletes have limited time to appropriately warm up and stretch. The soleus muscle is rarely involved, but it may be affected as well. Because it lies inferior to the gastrocnemius and originates posteriorly below the knee, the soleus muscle is more difficult to stretch and warm up.

Examination begins with visualization of the area, typically with the patient prone. Direct palpation of the calf muscle typically is painful. There also may be swelling or a defect noted. If the ankle plantarflexes when the examiner squeezes the calf, also known as the Thompson test, the Achilles tendon is functionally intact.[60] Some muscle tears involve enough fibers that the test may yield a positive result of decreased to no ankle plantar flexion. In all cases of calf pain, the Achilles tendon also should be evaluated and palpated for thickening, defect, and tenderness.

ROM and strength testing can be performed from the sitting position. With the knee flexed, assess the soleus muscle. With the knee extended, assess the gastrocnemius muscle. Test the patient's ability to bear weight as a way to monitor the patient's progress. MRI and diagnostic ultrasound may be useful in grading the injury or to assess for concomitant injury, but they typically are of limited use to make the diagnosis.[61]

Treatment consists of preventing shortening of the heel cord with a heel lift for a week or so. Longer period of time with a heel lift may produce a contracture of the gastroc soleus complex. Some patients feel better with a walking boot with a cam sole for the initial period. It is beneficial to start local ice, gentle stretching, and gentle massage of the area with or without an oral NSAID early. Formal physical therapy with the addition of modalities, such as electrical stimulation and ultrasound in conjunction with ROM techniques, proprioceptive and balance work, and progressive closed and open kinetic chain activities, also are helpful for return to athletics.[62] Most patients are able to resume prior activities within 6 weeks to 8 weeks.

PLANTAR FASCIITIS

Running and other sports, such as basketball, that demand repetitive weight-bearing activity on the feet, can lead to pain beneath the heel from inflammation or microtearing.[63] The plantar fascia is a thick ligamentous structure, which originates from the distal calcaneus, runs the course of the plantar arch, and inserts via fibrous bands into the proximal phalanx of each toe. The plantar fascia helps support the medial longitudinal arch of the foot and assist with ambulation. It has been proposed that its primary role is to dissipate the forces across the foot, which are primarily involved with heel strike and other loading conditions of the gait cycle. It also seems to have the capacity to store energy to be used to assist in propulsion.[63] Risk factors for plantar fasciitis include tightness of the heel cord, higher arch, and higher body mass index.[64] A combination of age and limited time for proper warming up also places weekend athletes at risk, for, as load increases the relative overuse, it leads to breakdown of the soft tissues, resulting in microtears at the origin of the plantar fascia. The repeated forces across the fascia create collagen breakdown and periostitis at the calcaneus, resulting in heel pain.

Patients often report relative increase in activity and present with sharp, knifelike pain about the heel. Due to the contracture of muscle tendon units in conjunction with bedrest, the initial steps out of bed in the morning are painful and improve with rest. The pain may worsen by the end of the day from extended period of standing.[65]

Patients can present with unilateral or bilateral symptoms. Examination reveals a tender plantar fascial insertion at the anteromedial calcaneus that worsens with ankle dorsiflexion.[66] The heel cord typically is contracted and may involve the gastrocnemius, soleus, or both muscles. Radiographs may reveal an associated calcaneal spur. Radiographs help to rule out occult fracture, arthritic changes, and tumor or avascular necrosis. Weight-bearing views are preferred. MRI and ultrasound rarely are needed to confirm a diagnosis, but they may be helpful if planning for surgery.[66] For those with persistent symptoms despite appropriate management, an electromyogram/nerve conduction study may be helpful to rule out nerve entrapment.

Treatment usually is nonoperative with rest, oral NSAIDs, local icing, injections, orthotics, and a good heel cord stretching program to include both the gastrocnemius and the soleus. A decrease in athletic participation by limiting activity for a few weeks to stay below the patient's threshold for pain symptoms with a gradual increase in frequency, duration, and intensity works well in the senior author's practice; 85% to 90% of plantar fasciitis is treated successfully without surgery.[67] Corticosteroid injections have been shown to have short-term improvements, but PRP injections have been shown to have better long-term improvements in comparison.[68] Corticosteroid injections also have the risk of fat pad atrophy and plantar fascia rupture.[69] Orthotics, such as heel wedges, shoe inserts, and night splints, have been utilized for decades with mixed results. They may provide short-term improvement in heel pain, but no long-term benefits found at 12-month follow-up.[70] Extracorporeal shock wave therapy also has been utilized, but it is expensive and the 6-month follow-up is near equal to placebo.[71] If there is failure of conservative management after 6 months to 12 months, surgical intervention can be considered.[72]

DISCLOSURE

The authors have nothing to disclose.

REFERENCES

1. Roberts DJ, Ouellet JF, McBeth PB, et al. The "weekend warrior": fact or fiction for major trauma? Can J Surg 2014;57(3):E62–8.
2. Mazzocca AD, Arciero RA, Bicos J. Evaluation and treatment of acromioclavicular joint injuries. Am J Sports Med 2007;35:316–29.
3. Li X, Ma R, Bedi A, et al. Management of acromioclavicular joint injuries. J Bone Joint Surg Am 2014;96(1):73–84.
4. Gorbaty JD, Hsu JE, Gee AO. Classifications in brief: rockwood classification of acromioclavicular joint separations. Clin Orthop Relat Res 2017;475(1):283–7.
5. Modi CS, Beazley J, Zywiel MG, et al. Controversies relating to the management of acromioclavicular joint dislocations. Bone Joint J 2013;95:1595–602.
6. Gokkus K, Saylik H, Atmaca ES, et al. Limited distal clavicle excision of acromioclavicular joint osteoarthritis. Orthop Traumatol Surg Res 2016;102(3):311–8.
7. Kim S, Blank A, Strauss E. Management of type 3 acromioclavicular joint dislocations–current controversies. Bull Hosp Joint Dis 2014;72(1):53–60.
8. Banaszek D, Pickell M, Wilson E, et al. Anatomical evaluation of the proximity of neurovascular structures during arthroscopically assisted acromioclavicular joint reconstruction: a cadaveric pilot study. Arthroscopy 2017;33:75–81.
9. Sirin E, Aydin N, Mert Topkar O. Acromioclavicular joint injuries: diagnosis, classification and ligamentoplasty procedures. EFORT Open Rev 2018;3(7):426–33.

10. Chang N, Furey A, Kurdin A. Operative versus nonoperative management of acute high-grade acromioclavicular dislocations: a systematic review and meta-analysis. J Orthop Trauma 2018;32(1):1–9.
11. Cutbush K, Hirpara KM. All-arthroscopic technique for reconstruction of acute acromioclavicular joint dislocations. Arthrosc Tech 2015;4:475–81.
12. Tempelhof S, Rupp S, Seil R. Age-related prevalence of rotator cuff tears in asymptomatic shoulders. J Shoulder Elbow Surg 1999;8:296–9.
13. Hermans J, Luime JJ, Meuffels DE, et al. Does this patient with shoulder pain have rotator fuff disease? The Rational Clinical Examination Systematic Review 2013;310(8):837–84.
14. Nazarian LN, Jacobson JA, Benson CB, et al. Imaging algorithms for evaluating suspected rotator cuff disease: Society of Radiologists in Ultrasound consensus conference statement. Radiology 2013;267(2):589–95.
15. Clement ND, Nie YX, McBirnie JM. Management of degenerative rotator cuff tears: a review and treatment strategy. Sports Med Arthrosc Rehabil Ther Technol 2012;4(1):48.
16. Lin MT, Chiang CF, Wu CH, et al. Comparative effectiveness of injection therapies in rotator cuff tendinopathy: a systematic review, pairwise and network meta-analysis of randomized controlled trials. Arch Phys Med Rehabil 2019;100(2): 336–49.
17. Finnoff JT, Smith J, Peck ER. Ultrasonography of the shoulder. Phys Med Rehabil Clin N Am 2010;21:481–507.
18. Okoroha K, Mehran N, Duncan J, et al. Characterization of rotator cuff tears: ultrasound versus magnetic resonance imaging. Orthopedics 2017;40:124–30.
19. Abechain JJK, Godinho GG, Matsunaga FT, et al. Functional outcomes of traumatic and non-traumatic rotator cuff tears after arthroscopic repair. World J Orthop 2017;8(8):631–7.
20. Tashjian RZ. AAOS clinical practice guideline: optimizing the management of rotator cuff problems. J Am Acad Orthop Surg 2011;19(6):380–3.
21. Thériault G, Lachance P. Golf injuries. Sports Med 1998;26(1):43–57.
22. Ciccotti MC, Schwartz MA. Diagnosis and treatment of medial epicondylitis of the elbow. Clin Sports Med 2004;23(4):693–705.
23. Pitzer ME, Seidenberg PH, Bader DA. Elbow tendinopathy. Med Clin North Am 2014;98(4):833–49.
24. Punam MD, Cohen M. Painful conditions about the elbow. Orthop Clin North Am 1999;30(1):109–18.
25. Vaquero-Picado A, Barco R, Antuña SA. Lateral epicondylitis of the elbow. EFORT Open Rev 2016;1(11):391–7.
26. Kachanathu SJ, Alenazi AM, Hafez AR, et al. Comparison of the effects of short-duration wrist joint splinting combined with physical therapy and physical therapy alone on the management of patients with lateral epicondylitis: a randomized clinical trial. Eur J Phys Rehabil Med 2019;55(4):488–93.
27. Xu Q, Chen J, Cheng L. Comparison of platelet rich plasma and corticosteroids in the management of lateral epicondylitis: a meta-analysis of randomized controlled trials. Int J Surg 2019;67:37–46.
28. Anderson D. Skier's thumb. Aust Fam Physician 2010;39(9):575–7.
29. Avery DM, Caggiano NM, Matullo KS. Ulnar collateral ligament injuries of the thumb: a comprehensive review. Orthop Clin North Am 2015;46(2):281–92.
30. Kozin SH, Bishop AT. Gamekeeper's thumb. Early diagnosis and treatment. Orthop Rev 1994;23(10):797–804.

31. Beutel BG, Melamed E, Rettig ME. The Stener lesion and complete ulnar collateral ligament injuries of the thumb: a review. Bull Hosp Jt Dis 2019;77(1):11–20.
32. Rocchi L, Merolli A, Morini A, et al. A modified spica-splint in postoperative early-motion management of skier's thumb lesion: a randomized clinical trial. Eur J Phys Rehabil Med 2014;50(1):49–57.
33. Sollerman C, Abrahamsson SO, Lundborg G, et al. Functional splinting versus plaster cast for ruptures of the ulnar collateral ligament of the thumb. A prospective randomized study of 63 cases. Acta Orthop Scand 1991;62(6):524–6.
34. Mahajan M, Rhemrev SJ. Rupture of the ulnar collateral ligament of the thumb - a review. Int J Emerg Med 2013;6(1):31.
35. Christensen T, Sarfani S, Shin AY, et al. Long-term outcomes of primary repair of chronic thumb ulnar collateral ligament injuries. Hand 2016;11(3):303–9.
36. Lee JC, Healy JC. Chapter 60 - sonography of muscle injury. Clinical ultrasound. 3rd edition 2011. p. 1137–57.
37. Pagorek S, Malone T. Principles of rehabilitation for muscle and tendon injuries. Physical rehab of the injured athlete. 4th edition 2012. p. 80–103.
38. Noehren B, Schmitz A, Hempel R, et al. Assessment of strength, flexibility, and running mechanics in men with iliotibial band syndrome. J Orthop Sports Phys Ther 2014;44(3):217–22.
39. Strauss EJ, Kim S, Calcei JG, et al. Iliotibial band syndrome: evaluation and management. J Am Acad Orthop Surg 2011;19(12):728–36.
40. Mitchell WG, Kettwich SC, Sibbitt WJ, et al. Outcomes and cost-effectiveness of ultrasound-guided injection of the trochanteric bursa. Rheumatol Int 2018;38(3):393–401.
41. Ali M, Oderuth E, Atchia I, et al. The use of platelet-rich plasma in the treatment of greater trochanteric pain syndrome: a systematic literature review. J Hip Preserv Surg 2018;5(3):209–19.
42. Figueroa D, Figuoeroa F, Calvo R. Patellar tendinopathy: diagnosis and treatment. J Am Acad Orthop Surg 2016;24(12):184–92.
43. Behzad H, Sharma A, Mousavizadeh R, et al. Mast cells exert pro-inflammatory effects of relevance to the pathophysiology of tendinopathy. Arthritis Res Ther 2013;15(6):184.
44. Zhang J, Wang JH. Production of PGE(2) increases in tendons subjected to repetitive mechanical loading and induces differentiation of tendon stem cells into non-tenocytes. J Orthop Res 2010;28(2):198–203.
45. Morton S, Williams S, Valle X, et al. Patellar tendinopathy and potential risk factors: an international database of cases and controls. Clin J Sport Med 2017;27(5):468–74.
46. Schwartz A, Watson JN, Hutchinson MR. Patellar tendinopathy. Sports Health 2015;7(5):415–520.
47. Filardo G, Di Matteo B, Kon E, et al. Platelet-rich plasma in tendon-related disorders: results and indications. Knee Surg Sports Traumatol Arthrosc 2018;26(7):1984–99.
48. Wang CJ. Extracorporeal shockwave therapy in musculoskeletal disorders. J Orthop Surg Res 2012;7:11.
49. Fox AJ, Wanivenhaus F, Burge AJ, et al. The human meniscus: a review of anatomy, function, injury, and advances in treatment. Clin Anat 2015;28(2):269–87.
50. Malanga GA, Nadler SF. Musculoskeletal physical examination: an evidence-based approach. 1st edition. Philadelphia: Elsevier; 2006. p. 306–11.
51. Thorlund JB, Pihl K, Nissen N, et al. Conundrum of mechanical knee symptoms: signifying feature of a meniscal tear? Br J Sports Med 2019;53:299–303.

52. Pujol N, Salle De Chou E, Boisrenoult P, et al. Platelet-rich plasma for open meniscal repair in young patients: any benefit? Knee Surg Sports Traumatol Arthrosc 2015;23:51–8.
53. Sihvonen R, Paavola M. Arthroscopic partial meniscectomy versus placebo surgery for a degenerative meniscus tear: a 2-year follow-up of the randomized controlled trial. Ann Rheum Dis 2018;77(2):188–95.
54. Bollen S. Epidemiology of knee injuries: diagnosis and triage. Br J Sports Med 2000;34(3):227–8.
55. Halinen J, Koivikko M, Lindahl J, et al. The efficacy of magnetic resonance imaging in acute multi-ligament injuries. Int Orthopedics 2009;33:1733–8.
56. Delee J, Drez D, Miller M. Orthopedic sports medicine: principles and practice. Philadelphia: Saunders; 2010. p. 1624–37.
57. Najibi S. The use of knee braces, Part 1: prophylactic knee braces in contact sports. Am J Sports Med 2005;33(4):602–11.
58. Fields K, Rigby M. Muscular calf injuries in runners. Curr Sports Med Rep 2016; 15(5):320–4.
59. Green B, Pizzari T. Calf muscle strain injuries in sport: a systematic review of risk factors for injury. Br J Sports Med 2017;51(16):1189–94.
60. Kor A. Dynamic techniques for clinical assessment of the athlete. Clin Podiatr Med Surg 2015;32(2):217–29.
61. Bright JM, Fields KB, Draper R. Ultrasound diagnosis of calf injuries. Sports Health 2017;9(4):352–5.
62. Sherry MA, Johnston TS, Heiderscheit BC. Rehabilitation of acute hamstring strain injuries. Clin Sports Med 2015;34(2):263–84.
63. Foye PM, Stitik TP, Sinha D. Physical medicine and rehabilitation for plantar fasciitis. Phys Med Rehabil 2010.
64. van Leeuwen KD, Rogers J, Winzenberg T, et al. Higher body mass index is associated with plantar fasciopathy/'plantar fasciitis': systematic review and meta-analysis of various clinical and imaging risk factors. Br J Sports Med 2016; 50(16):972–81.
65. Trojian T, Tucker AK. Plantar fasciitis. Am Fam Physician 2019;99(12):744–50.
66. Neufeld SK, Cerrato R. Plantar fasciitis: evaluation and treatment. J Am Acad Orthop Surg 2008;16(6):338–46.
67. Schepsis AA, Leach RE, Gorzyca J. Plantar fasciitis: etiology, treatment, surgical results, and review of the literature. Clin Orthop Relat Res 1991;266:185–96.
68. Shetty SH, Dhond A, Arora M, et al. Platelet-rich plasma has better long-term results than corticosteroids or placebo for chronic plantar fasciitis: randomized control trial. J Foot Ankle Surg 2019;58(1):42–6.
69. Kalaci A, Cakici H, Hapa O, et al. Treatment of plantar fasciitis using four different local injection modalities: a randomized prospective clinical trial. J Am Podiatr Med Assoc 2009;99(2):108–13.
70. Landorf KB, Keenan AM, Herbert RD. Effectiveness of foot orthoses to treat plantar fasciitis: a randomized trial. Arch Intern Med 2006;166(12):1305–10.
71. Kudo P, Dainty K, Clarfield M, et al. Randomized, placebo-controlled, double-blind clinical trial evaluating the treatment of plantar fasciitis with an extracorporeal shockwave therapy (ESWT) device: a North American confirmatory study. J Orthop Res 2006;24(2):115–23.
72. Thomas JL, Christensen JC, Kravitz SR, et al. The diagnosis and treatment of heel pain: a clinical practice guideline-revision 2010. J Foot Ankle Surg 2010;49(3): S1–19.

Geriatric Rehabilitation
Gait in the Elderly, Fall Prevention and Parkinson Disease

Randel Swanson, DO, PhD[a,b], Keith M. Robinson, MD[a,b],*

KEYWORDS

- Geriatrics • Rehabilitation • Aging • Deconditioning • Parkinsonism
- Durable medical equipment • Caregivers

KEY POINTS

- Aging-associated anatomic and physiologic decline begins during the fourth decade of life and progresses over the ensuing decades sometimes to a state of frailty, with the decline amplified when there is deconditioning.
- Aging-related gait and balance disorders leading to an increased risk of falling can be compensated for with the use of exercise interventions, durable medical equipment, and environmental modifications.
- Caregiver training is an essential component of geriatric rehabilitation.

WHAT IS GERIATRIC REHABILITATION?

Geriatric rehabilitation entails the application and expansion of standard rehabilitation tools and strategies to individuals who have achieved old age, defined chronologically as age 60 years and older. Normal aging is typically characterized by the synergistic decline of anatomic and physiologic reserve across organ systems, thus resulting in increasing disability with increasing age. For example, 22% of elderly women and 15% of elderly men depend on caregivers to perform basic self-care and mobility tasks, with 45.3% of those aged 75 years and older functionally disabled.[1,2] Geriatric rehabilitation assumes a multidisciplinary model of assessment and treatment to maximize function (self-care, mobility, communication) during aging and old age. Although uncomplicated conditions with minimal functional disability may be effectively treated by a single discipline, as the complexity of the conditions to be treated increases, the need for a multidisciplinary team becomes evident[3] (**Table 1**).

[a] Department of Physical Medicine and Rehabilitation, Perelman School of Medicine, University of Pennsylvania, Philadelphia, PA, USA; [b] Corporal Michael J. Crescenz Veterans Affairs Medical Center, 3800 Woodland Avenue, Philadelphia, PA 19104, USA
* Corresponding author.
E-mail address: Keith.Robinson@va.gov

Med Clin N Am 104 (2020) 327–343
https://doi.org/10.1016/j.mcna.2019.10.012
0025-7125/20/© 2019 Elsevier Inc. All rights reserved.
medical.theclinics.com

Table 1	
The multidisciplinary geriatric rehabilitation team	
Team Members	**Acronyms**
Physiatrist	PM&R
Physical therapist	PT
Occupational therapist	OT
Speech language pathologist	SLP
Nurse	RN
Social worker	SW
Neuropsychologist	NPsych
Behavioral specialist	BHS
Psychotherapist	Psych
Nutritionist	Nutr
Recreation therapist	RT
Prosthetist/orthotist	P/O

WHERE DOES GERIATRIC REHABILITATION OCCUR?

Medicare guidelines have driven the definitions of various levels of postacute care in which geriatric rehabilitation typically occurs, with settings ranging from acute inpatient rehabilitation (hospital level) to outpatient therapies. Admission and/or referral to postacute inpatient rehabilitation programs typically occurs after the event of illness, injury, and/or surgical procedures that necessitate acute hospitalization. Proactive discharge planning during the acute hospitalization becomes essential to support a shorter length of stay and to reduce iatrogenesis. It is expected that an older patient is assessed by the rehabilitation team during the acute hospital stay to define gaps between the older individual's prehospital functional status and current functional status, which may have declined during the event of illness/injury/inactivity. These gaps are then translated into a rehabilitation treatment plan that is matched with a posthospital rehabilitation level of care. Essentially, what occurs here is an extrapolation of the older patient's potential recovery and associated ability to tolerate different intensities of treatment at different levels of care based on the presence of a new impairment, such as a stroke, and that superimposes the effects of activity-induced deconditioning, concurrent chronic diseases, and normal aging.[4–8]

TREATMENT STRATEGIES IN GERIATRIC REHABILITATION

Treatment strategies that are exercise and cognitive remediation based can be characterized as either skilled or maintenance treatments.[3] Skilled rehabilitation is provided by physical therapy, occupational therapy, and speech therapy; is goal driven; and is insurance reimbursable as long a functional progress in response to treatment is documented, and annual spending caps are followed. These treatments are necessary in the event of acute illness (eg, pneumonia) or traumatic event (eg, a fall resulting in a femoral neck fracture) when inactivity is imposed. Maintenance rehabilitation is geared toward sustaining an optimal functional level over time, typically with regular exercise and cognitive activity that is self-directed or directed by caregivers, and usually self-funded; for example, hiring a fitness trainer or companion, or joining a group yoga or tai chi class.

Successful participation in rehabilitation presumes some relative integrity in systems of learning. Normal aging involves a decline in several aspects of learning, such as new skills acquisition, cognitive processing speed, and attention, particularly when sustained and/or divided. Learning takes longer, and more persistent repetition and sustained rehearsal during the acquisition of new cognitive and motor sequences are necessary. Rehabilitation treatment approaches must then be adapted behaviorally by the treatment team by creating conditions in which successful learning will occur. These conditions include[9]:

1. Contextualizing the learning of new skills in a manner that is meaningful to the individual experientially, and environmentally in which consistent cues are offered to reinforce successful task performance
2. Providing highly structured and organized treatment to minimize environmental distractions
3. Dissociating to-be-learned tasks into components, and then rebuilding these into meaningful, rational sequences
4. Applying communication strategies during treatment to compensate for visual and hearing losses; for example, speaking in a lower vocal pitch that accommodates high-frequency hearing loss, and enhancing verbal communication with gesturing, facial expressions, vocal inflection, and nonthreatening tactile contact
5. Operationalizing procedural learning strategies that are grounded in unconscious or implicit learning systems, that are more widely distributed in the brain, that are more dependent on learning how rather than learning what, and that use basic behavioral management approaches such as errorless learning

AGING-ASSOCIATED BIOLOGICAL CHANGES

Humans experience anatomic and physiologic decline beginning during the fourth decade of life (**Table 2**), and this decline is presumed irreversible. Normal aging is genetically programmed; however, random processes, such as exposure to environmental toxins and musculoskeletal wear and tear, may augment genetic programming. Genetic determinism of biological aging is reinforced by observations at the cellular level such as apoptosis or programmed cell death, and cellular senescence or the cessation of cellular mitotic divisions after a finite number of divisions occurring. Moreover, at the cellular level, damage occurs for an array of other reasons, including spontaneous genetic mutations and exposure to free radicals. Cellular damage is therefore thought to outstrip cellular repair, thus supporting the irreversibility of biological aging.[10,11]

Normal aging is nonparallel across organs systems and across individuals. Normal aging is associated with the acquisition of chronic diseases, and the relationship between normal aging and these diseases can be viewed along a spectrum with no interaction at one end, and with natural aging-related changes that become labeled as chronic diseases at the other end. The fundamental concept that underpins normal aging is that each organ system is viewed as having a decline in the reserve capacity; that is, compromised physiologic adaptability in response to stressors such as acute illness/injury and surgical procedures. Thus, recovery takes longer for older individuals compared with their younger counterparts, and recovery may be at more risk for being interrupted by medical instability and medical/surgical events.[10,11]

GERIATRIC FRAILTY

Geriatric frailty can be viewed as the cumulative and extreme effects of normal aging as superimposed by the negative effects of inactivity and multiple chronic diseases

Table 2
Major biological changes that occur during normal aging

Musculoskeletal, Including Joints and Bone	Sarcopenia with disproportionate loss of fast twitch/high force–producing muscle fibers; thinning of articular cartilage of joints; loss of elasticity of soft tissues; loss of bone mineral density
Neurologic	Decrease in speed of cognitive processing, mental flexibility, divided and sustained attention, and working memory; decrease in brain volume; decrease in motor reaction time; decline in accuracy of fine motor performance; degeneration on peripheral nerves; slower gait speed; decreased arm swing during walking; shortening of step length
Cardiovascular	Arterial wall thickening with compensatory increase in systolic blood pressure; thickening of left ventricular wall and stiffening of heart valves inducing lower myocardial oxygen consumption and heart rate responses during submaximal and maximal exercise efforts; slower responses to cardiovascular training effects during reconditioning and athletic training
Pulmonary	Decreased lung elasticity resulting in a decrease in chest wall excursion, lung volumes, and alveolar surface area for air exchange; sarcopenia of intercostal muscles with less energy-efficient breathing
Endocrine	Glucose intolerance; decline in growth hormone contributing to sarcopenia, bone mineral density loss, and immune compromise; estrogen depletion in women; decreased testosterone level in men
Immune	Decline in lymphocyte production, a weaker response of T cells to novel antigens, and weaker binding of B cells to antigens; heightening of inflammatory activation and increase in autoantibody levels
Gastrointestinal	Less efficient hepatic metabolism; colonic fibrosis
Genitourinary	Decrease in glomerular filtration rate in the kidneys with inefficient handling of fluids/electrolytes; reduction in renal perfusion, and number and size of nephrons; bladder fibrosis related to reduced capacity and urinary frequency; sarcopenia of urethral sphincter and pelvic floor muscles; prostatic hypertrophy, which may cause urethral obstruction in older men
Skin	Loss of hair pigment and skin wrinkling; loss in number and efficiency of sweat glands related to dry skin and inefficient thermoregulation
Special Senses	Decrease in lens accommodation of the eye resulting in compromised near vision or presbyopia; decrease in visual contrast and color discrimination, and slower visual adjustments during transitions from dim to bright environments; decrease in hearing of high-frequency sounds

(**Box 1**). Sarcopenia is a central component of geriatric frailty, and is hypothesized to result from dysregulation of neuromuscular, metabolic, and immune systems that induces upregulation of inflammatory responses in muscle tissue.[11,12]

DECONDITIONING IN THE ELDERLY

The deconditioning syndrome (**Table 3**) entails the negative anatomic and physiologic effects of inactivity and bed rest.[13,14] Sedentarism is epidemic among the elderly, related to lack of regular exercise participation or suboptimal exercise participation that does not counteract the effects of chronic inactivity, predisposing to the development of chronic illnesses such as diabetes mellitus, hyperlipidemia, coronary heart

> **Box 1**
> **Criteria for geriatric frailty**
>
> - More than 4.5 kg (10 pounds) weight loss or greater to or equal than 5% weight loss within 1 year
> - Subjective experience of exhaustion
> - Weakness as measured by compromised grip strength or by an inability to rise from a chair 5 times consecutively without use of the arms
> - Slow walking speed; that is, taking more than 6 seconds to walk 4.5 m (15 feet)
> - Decreased daily energy expenditure related to inactivity; that is, less than 383 kilocalories daily in men and less than 270 kilocalories daily in women
>
> The Cardiovascular Health Study index defines frailty if 3 of 5 criteria are met, whereas pre-frailty is defined by meeting 2 of the 5 criteria.

disease, obesity, and dementia. Survey data report that at least 50% of the current so-called baby boomer generation participate in no regular exercise.[15,16]

GENERAL EXERCISE PRESCRIPTION IN THE ELDERLY

While acknowledging a close interaction between normal aging and deconditioning, exercise interventions during rehabilitation are thought primarily to reverse and/or prevent deconditioning. Given aging-related sarcopenia, rehabilitation interventions are essential, including basic strengthening, functional mobility, gait and balance training, and self-care skills training. These motorically based treatments should

Table 3
The deconditioning syndrome

Musculoskeletal	Soft tissue and joint contracture; muscular atrophy causing weakness that may be more obvious in the proximal muscular groups; reduced repetitive muscular endurance; reduced bone mineral density
Neurologic	Delirium; sensory deprivation; impaired balance and coordination
Cardiovascular	Orthostasis; increased heart rate at rest and more rapid increase of heart rate with activity; increase of systolic blood pressure; reduced stroke volume and cardiac output; stasis of peripheral blood flow and increased blood coagulability
Pulmonary	Reduced lung volumes; increase in respiratory rate at rest and more rapidly with activity; inefficient clearance of secretions, including weaker coughing mechanism and less efficient ciliary activity predisposing to aspiration
Endocrine/Metabolic	Glucose intolerance; decreased androgen levels and spermatogenesis; disproportionate losses of nitrogen, calcium, sodium, and potassium
Gastrointestinal	Loss of appetite; atrophy of intestinal mucosa related to inefficient and slow absorption; inhibition of peristalsis related to constipation
Genitourinary	Incomplete bladder emptying related to increased risk of developing renal/bladder stones and urinary tract infections
Skin	Skin atrophy related to increase risk for developing pressure sores

be balanced with rational nutritional intake and environmental modifications designed to reduce falling risks and energy expenditure during self-directed daily life activities.

Regular exercise participation of at least 30 minutes at a moderate level of intensity at least 5 times weekly is recommended for reversing sedentarism and reducing risks for development of chronic illnesses. However, it is recognized that up to 75% of older Americans do not comply with this recommendation.[15,16] Regular exercise participation among the elderly can be challenging because of painful movement in weight-bearing joints, easier development of overuse tendinopathies, and sarcopenia that reduces achievable exercise intensity and muscular endurance during repetitive activities. Reduced aging-related cardiopulmonary reserve also impairs achievable exercise intensity. Guidelines for initiation of exercise programs in an elderly individual who does not have experience with habitual participation should follow the adage "start low and go slow," and include[5,12,16] (1) start with the lowest resistance band or weight possible that can be lifted 8 times before inducing muscular fatigue, then progress gradually to 15 repetitions before increasing the antigravity resistance or weight; (2) once the resistance is increased, start again at 8 repetitions and gradually increase again; (3) maintain a normal breathing pattern while performing the antigravity repetitions, exhaling while the resistance is pulled or while the weight is lifted; (4) repetitions should be slow, up to 3 seconds during the resistance phase (concentric muscle contraction) and up to 4 seconds during the recovery phase (eccentric muscle contraction); (5) joints and periarticular tissues should stay relaxed during movement; (6) muscular soreness should be expected during the early phases of initiating a strengthening program and should be distinguished from underlying exacerbations of muscle and joint diseases; (7) in addition to a strength training program, elderly individuals should aim for at least 30 min/d of walking/mobility for general cardiovascular health.

GAIT AND BALANCE ABNORMALITIES, AND FALLING, IN THE ELDERLY

Gait entails the sequential movements that occur during walking. When considering unilateral lower limb movement during walking, the gait cycle can be dissociated to several sequential components: lower limb swing (initial, then mid, then terminal) followed by lower limb stance (initial heel contact, then midfoot, then terminal push-off). Among individuals more than 70 years old, there is a 35% prevalence of gait abnormalities, with up to 50% of these associated with nonneurologic conditions. Normal aging is associated with several changes in gait, including postural flexion, reduced hip extension during terminal push-off, weak push-off related to less efficient ankle plantar flexors, and more variability in stride length.[17–19] In addition, certain gait abnormalities identified on clinical examination indicate an underlying pathologic process (**Table 4**).

The prevalence of balance difficulties among older adults is estimated to be up to 20%. As many as 25% of elderly individuals who have poor balance report unsafe participation in self-care activities, and up to 30% report that these preclude participation in activities such as exercise, social events, working, and driving. Balance or postural control involves attaining and then maintaining an upright position, as well as correcting posture when environmental conditions and sensory feedback are modified. Changes in balance associated with normal aging include increases in postural sway and reduced postural control, both of which are related to inefficient integration of the following systems: peripheral sensory, peripheral motor control, central attentional, and executive motor planning.[20–22]

Table 4
Clinical gait abnormalities that indicate a pathologic process

Gait Abnormality:	Potential Pathologic Process
Making efforts to limit unilateral weight bearing, along with reduction in step length and time in limb stance and leaning more to 1 side (antalgic gait)	Painful musculoskeletal structures such as knee osteoarthritis
Widening the base of feet support, excessive use of visual cueing, and loss of balance when visual cues are eliminated	Peripheral neuropathic process
Steppage gait	Compensation for a foot drop related to peroneal neuropathy causing weak ankle dorsiflexors
Circumduction unilaterally to compensate for spastic equinovarus ankle position (plantarflexed and externally rotated) during swing, then knee hyperextension in response to abnormal initial forefoot strike during stance	Unilateral brain injury/lesion such as a stroke, traumatic brain injury, or tumor
Lower limb scissoring and a stiff-legged pattern during bilateral lower limb swing	Cervical myelopathy
Excessive lateral sway with a wide base of support and an irregular step length	Cerebellar disease
Shuffling gait with festination and reduced arm swing, postural flexion and a narrow base of support, freezing	Parkinsonism

Falling is common among elderly individuals; its causes are multifactorial. About one-third of individuals who are more than 65 years old fall yearly, and about half of these individuals fall multiple times; 25% of falls result in moderate to severe injuries, including soft tissue bruising, lacerations, hip fractures, and concussions.[23] The best approach to understand the causes of falling is to consider the risk factors. Intrinsic risk factors include age greater than 80 years; orthostasis; recent history of falling; lower limb muscle weakness; gait/balance impairments; cognitive impairments, especially in focused and divided attention; depression; vision and hearing impairments; history of syncope, dizziness, parkinsonism, stroke, peripheral neuropathy; frailty; behavioral issues, such as impulsivity and poor judgment of safety; and fear of falling. Extrinsic risk factors include polypharmacy, particularly using antihypertensives, benzodiazepines, and sedatives; environmental hazards, such as slippery surfaces, stairs, poor lighting, unstable furniture, clutter, pets; ill-fitting clothing and footwear; and unfamiliar environments.

There are clinically accessible assessment tools of gait and balance that predict falling and that can be adapted in all assessment and treatment settings. The Timed Up and Go Test is a timed walking trial that entails an initial sit to stand from a chair with arm rests, then a walk out of 3 m (10 feet) with or without an assistive device, then a turnaround, then a walk back to the original destination, finally sitting down on the chair. Taking more than 12 seconds to complete this task is predictive of falling. The Short Physical Performance Battery encompasses a series of increasingly difficult motor tasks: side-by-side stance with feet together for 10 seconds (1 point if successful); tandem stance for 10 seconds (2 points); a timed 3-m (10-feet) walking speed test (4 points if performed in <3.62 seconds); and 5 repeated sit to stands within 1 minute

(4 points if performed in <11.19 seconds). A total score of less than 7 is highly predictive of falling. Slow walking speed is most predictive of higher falling risk in older women, and slow performance during repeated sit to stands is most predictive of higher falling risk in older men.[24–27]

The geriatric rehabilitation management of gait and balance impairments is multifactorial[23] and includes:

1. Secondary prevention regarding reduction of falling risk factors, including medication reduction, optimizing vision, and suggesting stable low-heeled footwear that provides total contact with the feet to enhance sensory feedback
2. Exercise programs that encompass core and proximal lower limb strengthening, repetitive muscular endurance training, cardiovascular training, gait/balance and coordination training; these programs include traditional physical therapies and group programs such as tai chi, dance, and yoga
3. Environment modifications to reduce recognized falling hazards, including home safety evaluations by physical and occupational therapists
4. Selection and safe use of appropriate assistive devices that provide enhanced sensory feedback

BASICS OF ASSISTIVE DEVICES AND ADAPTIVE EQUIPMENT

Seeking advice from the rehabilitation team can guide selection and safe use of assistive devices and adaptive equipment that encompass:

1. Mobility aids such as canes, walkers, crutches, and wheelchairs (**Table 5**)
2. Bathroom safety devices such as commodes, tub/shower chairs, tub transfer benches, raised toilet seats, and grab bars (**Table 6**)
3. Self-care devices such as reachers and built-up utensils (see **Table 6**)

These devices are intended to reduce energy expenditure during functional activities, provide compensatory proprioceptive feedback during essential survival skills, and create a safe physical environment for performing these skills as autonomously as possible.[6] Physical therapists typically are most knowledgeable about mobility devices and should be consulted when considering a manual wheelchair or power mobility (scooter or power wheelchair). Occupational therapists are most knowledgeable about bathroom safety devices and self-care devices, as well as power mobility. When considering the use of mobility devices, the weight-bearing status of all 4 limbs must be defined. For mobility devices, measurement of hand placement for canes, walkers, and crutches can be determined using the level parallel to greater the trochanter of the hip, and/or the level of the wrist crease in a fully extended upper limb; these approaches usually allow approximately 20° to 30° of elbow flexion. Mobility aids that are not properly fitted and inspected can increase falling risk. Self-purchase of such devices over the counter or borrowing them from family members and friends contributes to their unsafe use. Manual wheelchairs become necessary when lower limb weight bearing is not feasible because of severe lower extremity weakness or severely impaired balance. Manual wheelchairs can be either standard off-the-shelf items or customized and can be propelled either by the patient or by a caregiver. Power mobility (scooters and power wheelchairs) can be considered when the person's upper and lower limb motor control does not allow self-propulsion of a manual wheelchair. Cognitive functions must be fairly intact to support safe driving and manipulation of the power accessories and components. A driving safety test, and sometimes driver's training, are essential.

Table 5 Mobility aids		
Canes	Single-point cane Quad cane Hemicane	Do not provide antigravity support Require full weight bearing of all limbs Held in hand/arm opposite from the weaker side During gait cycle, advanced with the weaker lower limb
Walkers	Standard walker (no wheels) 2-wheeled rolling walker (front wheels) 4-wheeled rolling walker	Provide some antigravity support Need intact upper limb and trunk motor control Standard walker is appropriate when the gait pattern is nonfluid or step-to, as in poststroke hemiparesis 2-wheeled walkers require a more continuous and fluid gait pattern; appropriate for indoor use 4-wheeled walkers with hand brakes require a fluid gait pattern for safe use, can be used indoors and outdoors, and often have a seating system built in to allow seated rest breaks
Crutches	Axillary crutches Forearm crutches	Require good upper limb strength and motor control Axillary crutches demand a high level of dynamic standing balance, are typically used when weight bearing is restricted temporarily, and require a swing-to gait on 1 limb Forearm crutches are intended for long-term use and are best used bilaterally; a fluid gait pattern is required
Wheelchairs	Standard manual wheelchairs Custom manual wheelchairs	Necessary when lower limb weight bearing is not feasible because of severe weakness or impaired balance Custom manual wheelchairs are individualized to meet the needs of the patient, including recline and tilt in space options Both can encompass an array of components, including foot/leg/arm rests and various seating options Typically designed to have anterior casters and large posterior wheels with rims that can be used to self-propel with the upper limbs (can lead to repetitive overuse syndromes of the shoulder) Lightweight travel/transport wheelchairs are not self-propelled

(continued on next page)

Table 5 (continued)		
Power Mobility	Scooters Power wheelchairs	Considered when upper and lower limb motor control does not allow self-propulsion of a manual wheelchair, when walking endurance cannot be sustained, or when increased autonomy of mobility is sought Cognitive functions must be intact to support safe driving and manipulation of the power accessories and components Driving safety test and/or driver's training are essential Scooters: used for community mobility, not within the home; 3 or 4 wheeled; require good sitting balance given unsupportive seating systems for postural support Power wheelchairs: used for total mobility (inside/outside the home); drive controls can be front, mid or rear wheeled; steering typically involves using a toggle or joystick unilaterally by the upper limb that has better motor control; custom seating options available, including to accommodate poor sitting balance

Several environmental modifications can be considered to support safer mobility, particularly when negotiating nonlevel surfaces such as stairs. Safety railings either unilaterally or bilaterally on stairways can allow the upper limbs to compensate for weak lower limbs, and for compromised balance. Stair glides entail an electrically powered seat attached to a track that can arise or descend a stairway while the person is seated. A safe and autonomous transfer or one that is guided by a caregiver is essential for safe use of stair glides. Medicare funding for mobility devices tends to favor the use of the least restrictive device that can support safe transfers and walking. For example, selection of a walker rather than a cane must be clinically justified, and purchase of concurrent mobility aids, such as both a walker and a wheelchair, usually is not funded by Medicare. In persons who are homebound, a home environmental evaluation by both a physical therapist and an occupational therapist can be performed, and recommendations can be made to modify and/or embellish the environment with durable medical equipment and adaptive devices that facilitate safer and energy-efficient execution of daily survival skills, and reduce falling risks. Medicare typically does not pay for bathroom safety devices and self-care adaptive equipment, with the exception of commodes.

REHABILITATION OF PARKINSON DISEASE

Parkinson disease encompasses distinct involuntary motor signs, including tremor, bradykinesia or slow movement, trunk and limb rigidity, low volume of speech output,

Table 6
Bathroom safety devices and self-care adaptive equipment

Bedside Commodes	Can be used to accommodate nighttime toileting to avoid unsafe excursions
	Frames without the collection pan can be used over bathroom toilet to serve as elevated toilet seat and support a safer transfer on/off the toilet
Raised Toilet Seat	Can be directly secured to the base of the toilet
	Provides a higher base of support for a safer toilet transfer
Shower/tub chair	Allow sitting during showering when standing endurance and/or safety during standing on the wet and slippery tub or shower floor is problematic
Transfer Benches	Placed in the posterior of the tub
	Allows a seated rotational and scooting-type transfer across the bench that sits inside the tub, as well as sitting during showering
Hand-held Shower Devices	Preferred as the source of water when seated during showering
Grab Bars	Can be strategically placed on the wall inside the shower or on the wall surrounding the tub or toilet to support safe transfers
	Grab bars should be attached to the wall using hardware that can be secured to studs inside of the wall
Self-care Adaptive Equipment	Includes reachers, built-up handles on utensils, rocker knives to cut or chop food when there is functional use of only 1 upper limb, sock donners, and buttonholing devices

shuffling gait, balance dysfunction, and motor blocks or freezing. Although bradyphrenia, or slowness of thinking, also is a common cognitive feature, the dementia associated with Parkinson disease usually occurs later in the clinical course and typically entails poor initiation of activities as well as memory loss, language deficits, and executive dysfunction.[28] Animal model studies have supported that exercise is neuroprotective in Parkinson disease by stimulation of dopamine synthesis in the brain. Several principles can be articulated that emerge from a robust observational literature in humans that supports the application of rehabilitation treatments in Parkinson disease[29–31]:

1. Environmental and contextual factors, specifically applying external visual and auditory cueing systems, enhance motor control, gait, and balance
2. Internal perception of speech output and motor control can be modified to enhance vocal volume, and restricted movements, respectively, by applications of treatments grounded in the work of Ramig and colleagues[32] known as Lee Silverman Voice Treatment (LSVT)/LOUD, to treat hypokinetic dysarthria, and LSVT/BIG, to treat movement restricted by bradykinesia and rigidity[33]
3. Exercise-based treatment interventions should be initiated when the disease severity is mild
4. Although it cannot be firmly established when rehabilitation interventions are no longer beneficial, caregivers must be involved in all aspects of treatment, and, at times, the focus of treatment, particularly when the disease is severe and/or at a later stage
5. Loss reactions and depression should be explored as confounders of a patient's clinical presentation, as related to an array of factors associated with the disease

trajectory, including premature retirement, compromised physical and social role competence, and feeling stigmatized by the disease

6. Pain and fatigue should be recognized as treatment confounders; musculoskeletal pain, such as that generated from osteoarthritis and rigid soft tissues, makes functional movements stressful to joints and musculoskeletal soft tissues, and effortful, resulting in expenditure of more energy during routine movements and resulting in easier fatigability; painful dystonia as a side effect of dopaminergic agents is an idiosyncratic pain generator in Parkinson disease

Exercise interventions should be performed when the individual is in the on-medication state. Rigorously studied exercise-based interventions to treat gait and balance difficulties in Parkinson disease are those that have applied external visual and auditory cueing systems that enhance visuospatial and temporal influences on motor control. The application of sensory cueing is grounded in a hypothesis that there is impairment internally of the integration of proprioceptive information that directs motor control, thus inducing flexed posture, and a poorly timed, nonfluid gait pattern. External sensory cueing is viewed as a bypass strategy that may engage alternative neural networks to guide motor control. External visual and auditory cueing provides on-line compensatory feedback to support upright stance and better timing and fluidity of gait.[34] Commonly applied visual cues have included floor stripes, timed lighting, and mirrors, and commonly applied auditory cues have included music and metronomes. Clinical investigation has shown that gait velocity and walking speed were consistently but not universally improved under the cued conditions. Visual cues were more consistently observed to improve stride length, whereas auditory cues were observed to improved cadence. Sensory cues that were presented unpredictably were detrimental by disallowing engagement of internal cueing systems necessary for anticipation of movement initiation. One hypothesis generated to explain the effectiveness of external cueing is that they are compensating for a defective internal timekeeper in people who have Parkinson disease.[34–36]

Up to 70% of individuals who have Parkinson disease fall yearly, and up to 13% fall more than once weekly, and falling-associated injuries are twice as common as in the general elderly population and more frequent than in those who have neurodegenerative disease without parkinsonian features. Although there are falling risk factors that may be obvious in Parkinson disease, including gait and balance problems; cognitive difficulties such as compromised motor planning; and fear of falling when recurrent falls are experienced, several of these risk factors are idiosyncratic to this neurodegenerative process, including autonomic dysfunction, dopaminergic medication side effects such as hallucinations and dyskinesias, and freezing of gait or motor blocks. Multidimensional risk factor modification in combination with exercise interventions, the use of compensatory assistive devices, and environmental modifications, as similarly applied in the general elderly population, have been proposed as a rational model to reduce falling risks and events among those who have Parkinson disease, as well as recognizing that the idiosyncratic risk factors can be targeted for modification.[37,38]

Freezing of gait is a poorly understood phenomenon; it is difficult to investigate clinically given its unpredictability; it is usually considered refractory to dopaminergic medications. It is common in Parkinson disease and associated with more severe and later-stage disease. Freezing of gait has been categorized syndromically as to where it commonly occurs: start hesitation; gait arrests when approaching objects such as a chair; gait arrests when contained within narrow spaces such as doorways; gait arrests during turning; and hesitations when walking in open spaces. What seems to be a common feature about most of these categories is that a motor program must either be initiated or modified to sustain continuous walking through time and space. What empirically has been viewed as variably effective is when proprioceptive feedback is modified, as by the use of a 4-wheeled walker that may provide more enhanced and consistent proprioceptive feedback, and an externally generated behavioral strategy that requires that the individual stop, momentarily relax in static stance, then reinitiate the gait cycle by disconnecting the "glued" feet from the ground by hyperflexing the hip and knee of the initiating limb in a manner of stepping out and over a real (such as provided in some commercially available rollators that can trigger a laser beam) or imagined visual cue on the ground. Such a strategy can be taught procedurally to patients who freeze and their caregivers.[39–41]

TREATMENT OF HYPOKINETIC DYSARTHRIA AND PARKINSONIAN RIGIDITY USING PERCEPTUAL RETRAINING

Hypokinetic dysarthria is related to rigidity and bradykinesia of laryngeal and respiratory muscles, thus inducing low vocal volumes and speech unintelligibility. What is hypothesized to occur over time is that the individuals who have hypokinetic dysarthria internally modify their own feedback or self-monitoring systems of speech output, resulting in a perception that the low-volume speech pattern is normal.[32,42,43]

The best-studied behaviorally based treatment is LSVT, or LSVT/LOUD, an exercise-based speech therapy that increases strength and sustained muscular endurance of the respiratory muscles in order to generate a greater respiratory effort to overcome the rigidity of the laryngeal muscles that creates resistance to airflow to support adequate vocal volume. Moreover, it facilitates more complete vocal cord adduction, and recalibrates the internal acoustic perception of the person's own speech output. This treatment should be performed by speech therapists who are certified. Practice is required during and after completion of treatment to sustain gains made during and after exposure to this intensive intervention, and reported outcomes include improved vocal volume, vocal intelligibility, use of facial expression during speech output, and swallowing given the overlap of muscles used that control speech and swallowing.[32,43,44]

LSVT/BIG is a physical and/or occupational therapy approach that has extrapolated the concepts developed by LSVT to treat limb and trunk rigidity and bradykinesia as cardinal features of Parkinson disease. This intensive treatment uses repetitive movements that are high amplitude and demonstrative with the intent to counteract patients' proprioceptive sense that contributes to the restrictive movement patterns that occur with Parkinson disease and that result in a misperception of normal and fluid movement.[33]

CAREGIVER TRAINING

Caregivers have been categorized as either formal or informal. Formal caregivers provide personal care services that are purchased, whereas informal caregivers provide these services without pay and within the boundaries of familial and/or intimate relationships. Purchase of formal caregivers can be expensive, thus most elderly disabled patients depend on informal caregivers, broadly defined as spouses, adult children/grandchildren, other extended family members, friends, neighbors, and church/volunteer association members. Caregivers determine whether continued life in the least restrictive community-based residential setting is realistic and safe for the elderly disabled individual. Caregivers spend on average up to 20 hours weekly providing care including toileting, mobility assistance, dysphagia management, meal preparation, shopping, and transportation; more hours of service are provided by cohabitating dyads.[45,46] The saying that knowledge is power serves as the basic assumption when the rehabilitation team interacts with the patient-caregiver dyad: advise on durable medical equipment and environmental modifications; support emotionally; provide resource information; teach maintenance exercise, cognitive remediation, and incontinence management strategies; and counsel on behavioral management of difficult behaviors. It should be recognized that caregiver training may contribute even more to caregiver strain in that the demands placed on the caregiver may be heightened, necessitating an increase in the hours of service provision to perform additional duties.

Because caregivers define the interpersonal and physical environments in which cognitively impaired and/or disabled elderly individuals live, several factors focusing on the abilities of caregivers to create meaningful environment should be considered[28]: (1) the caregiver's own cognitive functions, emotional stability, and functional status (ie, does the caregiver also have dementia, depression, physical disability?); (2) the quality of the caregiver's relationship with the disabled individual (ie, is there long-standing tension/abuse exacerbated by relationship asymmetries?); (3) exhaustion (is the unpaid/informal caregiver concurrently employed outside of the home to generate necessary income; is the caregiver sleep deprived because of nighttime duties that include toileting and linen changes if there is incontinence?); (4) is there caregiver burnout (ie, is the caregiver receptive to suggestions by the rehabilitation team to modify the environment and/or practice novel treatment strategies and home exercise programs)?

Several basic tenets of behavioral management should be offered to the caregivers of geriatric patients[28]:

1. Create structured daily routines that are predictable, consistent, balanced, and that minimize distractions and allow rest breaks
2. Reward desired, positive, productive behaviors using communication skills that offer reinforcement, including verbal praise, smiling, and nonthreatening touch
3. Respond to undesired and counterproductive behaviors (anger, aggression, impulsivity) neutrally, and then attempt redirection away from possible environmental triggers of such behaviors
4. Survey the internal and external environments, respectively, of the patient, to define triggers that precipitate difficult behaviors, including pain, hunger, anxiety, depression, paranoia, fear, as well as sensory overload and perceived interpersonal threat

An array of geriatric caregiver training programs has been promoted and investigated when the patient-caregiver dyad must manage a dementia. These programs include nursing-driven cognitive-behavioral approaches designed to counteract caregiver depression using learned optimism and supporting the caregivers to re-engage their inner locus of control to counteract the sense of being controlled by outer forces.[47,48] In addition, risk factor modification to address caregiver strain should be pursued: treatment of depression; sleep regulation; staying socially connected to the caregiver's own support systems.[49]

Among the best operationalized caregiver training programs is one that is home based, provided by occupational therapists, and that was investigated by Gitlin and colleagues[50,51] as part of the National Institutes of Health Resources for Enhancing Alzheimer's Caregiver Health (REACH) initiative, the Environmental Skill Building program. The goal here is to reduce the disparity between personal competence of the caregiver and the environmental demands on the caregiver.

DISCLOSURE

Neither Dr R. Swanson nor Dr K.M. Robinson have commercial or financial conflicts of interest or funding sources.

REFERENCES

1. Weber DC, Fleming KC, Evans JM. Rehabilitation of geriatric patients. Mayo Clin Proc 1995;70:1198–204.
2. Manini T. Development of physical disability in older adults. Curr Aging Sci 2011; 4:184–91.
3. Robinson KM. Assessing function. In: Forciea MA, Lavizzo-Mourey R, Schwab EP, editors. Geriatric secrets. 2nd edition. Philadelphia: Hanley and Belfus, Inc.; 2000. p. 121–8.
4. Hoenig H, Colon-Emeric C. Overview of geriatric rehabilitation: patient assessment and indications for rehabilitation. In: Schmader KE, Givens J, editors. Wolters Kluwer; 2019. Available at: https://www.uptodate.com/contents/overview-of-geriatric-rehabilitation-patient-assessment.
5. Needham DM. Mobilizing patients in the intensive care unit: improving neuromuscular weakness and physical function. JAMA 2008;300:1685–90.
6. Hoenig H, Cary M. Overview of geriatric rehabilitation: program components and settings for rehabilitation. In: Schmader KE, Givens J, editors. UpToDate. Wolters Kluwer; 2019. Available at: https://www.uptodate.com/contents/overview-of-geriatric-rehabilitation program components.
7. Jeng G, Tinetti ME. The journeyacross the health care (dis)continuum for vulnerable patients: policies, pitfalls and possibilities. JAMA 2012;307:2157–8.
8. Yurkofsky M, Ouslander JG. Medical care in skilled nursing facilities. In: Schmader KE, Givens J, editors. UpToDate. Wolters Kluwer; 2019. Available at: https://www.uptodate.com/contents/medical-care-in-skilled-nursing-facilities-snfs-in-the-united-states.
9. Robinson KM, Grossman M. Rehabilitation of dementia. In: Selzer ME, Clarke S, Cohen LG, et al, editors. Textbook of neural repair and rehabilitation. Cambridge (United Kingdom): Cambridge University Press; 2006. p. 488–511.
10. Ljubunicic P, Reznick A. The evolutionary theories of aging revisited—a mini-review. Gerontology 2009;55:205–16.
11. Fedarko N. The biology of aging and frailty. Clin Geriatr Med 2011;27:27–37.
12. Fried LP, Tangen CM, Walston J, et al. Frailty in older adults: evidence for a phenotype. J Gerontol A Biol Sci Med Sci 2001;56:M146–56.
13. Gill TM, Allore H, Guo Z. The deleterious effects of bed rest among community-living elderly persons. J Gerontol A Biol Sci Med Sci 2004;59A:M755–61.
14. Vorhies D, Riley DE. Deconditioning. Clin Geriatr Med 1993;9:745–83.
15. Morey MC. Physical activity and exercise in older adults. In: Schmader KE, Givens J, editors. UpToDate. Wolters Kluwer; 2019. Available at: https://uptodate.com/contents/physical-activity-and exercise-in-older-adults.
16. National Center for Health Statistics. Healthy people 2010: final review. Hyattsville (MD): PHS Publication number: 2012-1038; 2012.
17. Verghese J, LeValley A, Hall CB, et al. Epidemiology of gait disorders in community-residing adults. J Am Geriatr Soc 2006;54:255–61.
18. Oh-Park M. Interplay between cognition and mobility in older adults. Annals of Geriatric Medicine and Research 2017;21:2–9.

19. Brach JS, Vanswearingen JM. Interventions to improve walking in older adults. Curr Transl Geriatr Exp Gerontol Rep 2014;2. https://doi.org/10.1007/s13670-013-0059-0. Available at: https://www.ncbi.nih.gov/pubmed23419641.
20. Noohu MM, Dey AB, Hussain ME. Relevance of balance measurement tools and balance training for fall prevention in older adults. Journal of Clinical Gerontology and Geriatrics 2014;5:31–5.
21. Frank JS, Horak FB, Nutt J. Centrally initiated postural control adjustments in Parkinsonian patients on and off levodopa. J Neurophysiol 2000;84:2440–8.
22. Lin HW, Bhattacharyya N. Balance disorders in the elderly: epidemiology and functional impact. Laryngoscope 2012;122:1858–61.
23. Gillespie L, Robertson W, Gillespie C, et al. Interventions for preventing falls in older people living in the community. Cochrane Database Syst Rev 2012;(9):CD007146.
24. Barry E, Galvin R, Keogh C, et al. Is the Timed Up and Go test a useful predictor of risk of falls in community dwelling older adults: a systemic response and meta-analysis? BMC Geriatr 2014;14:14.
25. Vasunilashorn SM, Coppin AK, Patel KV, et al. Use of short physical performance battery to predict loss of ability to walk 400 meters: analysis from the InCHIANTI study. J Gerontol A Biol Sci Med Sci 2009;64:223–9.
26. Shumway-Cook A, Brauer S, Woollacott M. Predicting the risk of falls in community-dwelling older adults using the timed up and go test. Phys Ther 2000;80:896–903.
27. Guralnick JM, Rerrucci L, Somonsick EM, et al. Lower extremity function in persons over the age of 70 years old as a predictor of subsequent disability. N Engl J Med 1995;332:556–61.
28. Robinson KM, Traweek LS. Rehabilitation after deep brain stimulation. In: Baltuch GH, Stern MB, editors. Deep brain stimulation for Parkinson's disease. New York: Informa Healthcare; 2007. p. 139–86.
29. Sutoo D, Akiyama K. Regulation of brain function by exercise. Neurobiol Dis 2003;13:1–14.
30. Tillerson JL, Caudle WM, Reveron ME, et al. Exercise induces behavioral recovery and attenuates neurochemical deficits in rodents models of Parkinson disease. Neuroscience 2003;119:899–911.
31. Montgomery EB. Rehabilitation approaches to Parkinson disease. Parkinsonism Relat Disord 2004;10:S43–7.
32. Ramig LO, Fox C, Sapir W. Parkinson disease: speech and voice disorders and their treatment with Lee Silverman Voice Treatment. Semin Speech Lang 2004;25:169–80.
33. Fox C, Ebers G, Ramig L, et al. LSVT LOUD and LSVT BIG: behavioral treatment programs for speech and body movement in Parkinson disease. Parkinsons Dis 2012;39:391146.
34. Rubinstein TC, Giladi N, Hausdorff JM. The power of cueing to circumvent dopamine deficits: a review of physical therapy treatment of gait disturbances in Parkinson's disease. Movement Disord 2002;17:1148–60.
35. Azulay JP, Mesure S, Amblard B, et al. Visual control of locomotion. Brain 1999;122:111–20.
36. Dietz V. Gait disorders in spasticity and Parkinson disease. Adv Neurol 2001;87:143–54.
37. Wielinski CL, Erickson-Davis C, Wichman R, et al. Falls and injuries resulting from falls among patients with Parkinson's disease and other Parkinsonian syndrome. Movement Disord 2005;20:721–5.

38. Robinson KM, Dennison AC, Roalf D, et al. Falling risk factors in Parkinson disease. NeuroRehabilitation 2005;20:169–82.
39. Giladi N, Treves A, Simon ES, et al. Freezing of gait in patients with advance Parkinson's disease. J Neural Transm 2001;108:53–61.
40. Schaafsma JD, Balash Y, Gurevich T, et al. Characterization of freezing of gait subtypes and the response of each to levodopa in Parkinson's disease. Eur J Neurol 2003;10:391–8.
41. Cubo E, Moore CG, Leurgans S, et al. Wheeled and standard walkers in Parkinson's disease patients with freezing of gait. Parkinsonism Relat Disord 2003; 10:9–14.
42. Goberman AM, Coehlo C. Acoustic analysis of Parkinsonian speech I: speech characteristics and L-dopa therapy. NeuroRehabilitation 2002;17:237–46.
43. Ramig LO, Sapir S, Countryman S, et al. Intensive voice treatment (LSVT®)for patients with Parkinson's disease: a 2 year follow up study. J Neurol Neurosurg Psychiatry 2001;71:493–8.
44. Spielman JI, Borod JC, Ramig LO. The effects of intensive voice treatment on facial expressiveness in Parkinson disease. Cogn Behav Neurol 2003;16:177–8.
45. National Alliance for Caregiving, American Association of Retired People. Caregiving in the US 2009. Available at: https://assets.aarp.org/rgcenter/il/caregiving_09_fr.pdf.
46. National Alliance for Caregiving, American Association of Retired People. A focused look at those caring for someone age 50 or older: companion report to caregiving in the US: executive Summary 2009. Available at: https://assets.aarp.org/rgcenter/il/caregiving_09_fr/pdf.
47. Habermann B. Spousal perspective of Parkinson' disease in middle life. J Adv Nurs 2000;31:14091415.
48. Lyons KS, Stewart BJ, Archbold PG, et al. Pessimism and optimism as early warning signs of compromised health for caregivers of patients with Parkinson's disease. Nurs Res 2004;53:354–62.
49. Trend P, Kaye J, Gage H, et al. Short-term effectiveness of intensive multidisciplinary rehabilitation for people with Parkinson's disease and their carers. Clin Rehabil 2002;16:717–25.
50. Gitlin LN, Hauck WW, Dennis MP, et al. Maintenance of the effects of the home environmental skill-building program for family caregivers and individuals with Alzheimer's disease and related disorders. J Gerontol A Biol Sci Med Sci 2005; 60A:368–74.
51. Gitlin LN, Winter L, Corcoran M, et al. Effects of the home environmental skill building-on the caregiver-care recipient dyad: 6-month outcomes from the Philadelphia REACH initiative. Gerontologist 2003;43:532–46.

Determination of Postacute Hospitalization Level of Care

Robert Samuel Mayer, MD, MEHP[a],*, Amira Noles, MD[a],
Dominique Vinh, MD, MBA[b]

KEYWORDS

- Inpatient rehabilitation • Skilled nursing facility • Long-term acute care hospital
- Rehabilitation outcomes • Stroke rehabilitation • Amputation care
- Hip fracture rehabilitation

KEY POINTS

- Multiple levels of rehabilitation care exist in the United States, including inpatient rehabilitation facilities (IRFs), skilled care facilities (SNFs), long-term acute care (LTAC) hospitals, home health agencies (HHA), and outpatient rehabilitation (OP).
- Each level of care has specific admission criteria and various payment incentives to control costs.
- Outcomes vary among levels of care, depending on the diagnosis and functional status of the patient.
- An interdisciplinary team can best decide the appropriate level of rehabilitation care after an acute hospitalization.

INTRODUCTION

One of the most challenging aspects of physical medicine and rehabilitation is the determination of the appropriate level of rehabilitation care for a given patient, especially following an acute hospitalization. In the United States, we are blessed with many options for postacute care:

- Inpatient rehabilitation facilities (IRFs),
- Long-term acute care (LTAC) hospitals,
- Skilled nursing facilities (SNFs),

[a] Department of Physical Medicine and Rehabilitation, Johns Hopkins University School of Medicine, 600 North Wolfe Street, Phipps 174, Baltimore, MD 21287, USA; [b] Department of Physical Medicine and Rehabilitation, Johns Hopkins University School of Medicine, 5505 Hopkins Bayview Circle, Baltimore, MD 21224, USA
* Corresponding author.
E-mail address: rmayer2@jhmi.edu
Twitter: @rsmayer2 (R.S.M.)

Med Clin N Am 104 (2020) 345–357
https://doi.org/10.1016/j.mcna.2019.10.011
0025-7125/20/© 2019 Elsevier Inc. All rights reserved.

- Home health agencies (HHA), and
- Outpatient rehabilitation (OP).

Each of these levels of care have distinct criteria for admission, payment methodologies, resources, advantages, and disadvantages. There can be some overlap among these levels of care, and choosing an appropriate level of care for a given patient often involves significant professional judgment. In this article, we review factors in this decision-making process and describe each level of care. We also provide some data on comparative outcomes.

PATIENT EVALUATION

An interdisciplinary team of health care professionals should evaluate the patient during his/her acute hospitalization to assess their rehabilitation needs and potential. Involvement of the patient and family in decision making is critical. Rehabilitation is not something done *to* a patient; it is done *with* a patient, and the patient's motivation and goals are critical in this determination. One cannot overemphasize the role of social support in assessment. The team needs to determine where the patient will likely go after rehabilitation is complete, and whether discharge to a community setting is possible. This must take into account not only the patient's disability, but also the availability of caregivers and how the patient may manage environmental barriers (eg, stairs) that are present in the patient's home. Furthermore, the team must act as prognosticators, and make informed guesses on the patient's progress with future rehabilitation.

The interdisciplinary team consists of rehabilitation therapists (physical therapy, occupational therapy, and/or speech pathology), nursing, social work, the primary medical team, and consulting physiatrists. Each team member has a distinct role in this process. Rehabilitation therapists determine the patient's current functional status and assess the patient's ability to tolerate therapies. Specifically, physical therapy assesses mobility, occupational therapy assesses self-care, and speech pathology assesses communication, cognition, and swallowing. Nursing assesses bowel and bladder function, nutrition, and specialized treatments (eg, intravenous medication, respiratory therapy, and wound care). Importantly, they assess the patient's impairment during "off" hours when other staff are usually not there (eg, "sun-downing" at night). Social workers address the patient's home environment for physical and social barriers to discharge, and help determine the availability of caregiver support. The primary medical team caring for the patient in the hospital must determine when the patient is medically stable for discharge, and what follow-up treatments are needed after the patient leaves. The physiatrist will reconcile these elements together, and determine the patient's functional prognosis. Furthermore, the physiatrist needs to assess whether the postacute facility can manage the patient's ongoing needs safely.

Key questions the team must answer are:

- What are the patient's goals for rehabilitation?
- Can the patient realistically achieve these goals?
- Does the patient have the motivation to participate in an intensive rehabilitation program?
- How much therapy can the patient tolerate due to endurance or pain?
- Can anything be done to improve the patient's therapy tolerance?
- What are the patient's ongoing medical needs? How much nursing and physician care will be required during rehabilitation?

- Will the patient require around-the-clock supervision or assistance after rehabilitation is complete?
- If so, are caregivers able to provide this assistance?
- Does the patient's home have environmental barriers, such as stairs or narrow doorways? If so, can the patient overcome these barriers?

In the United States. there is a yet another stakeholder that plays a crucial role in this process—the third-party payor. Unless the patient has substantial financial resources, either a commercial insurance or a government program (Medicare, Medicaid, and Veterans Administration) will bear the expense, and will determine whether to fund any proposed rehabilitation program. Although third-party payors do not directly determine care, they do determine payment, which may effectively nullify any recommendations made by the patient's care team. In general, commercial insurance will make this determination prospectively through previous authorization. Government programs will generally make retrospective audits, and possibly deny payment for services after they are rendered. Government programs offer transparency in their admission criteria, which are publicly available online (ie, the Center for Medicare and Medicaid Services Web site: cms.gov). Commercial insurance often mirrors these guidelines, but may be more opaque in their interpretation. They often use proprietary vendor guidelines (Millman and Interqual are the 2 largest of these proprietors). Insurances may also have specific benefit limitations on individual policies, for example, limits on the number of therapy visits in a year, or whether they will pay for long-term acute hospitalization. For the purposes of this article, however, we describe the Medicare criteria for each level of care, keeping in mind that other payors may not honor these.

LEVELS OF REHABILITATION CARE

Table 1 lists levels of rehabilitation care available in the United States from most intensive to least intensive. Each level of care also varies in the intensity of nursing services and the frequency and specialization of physician and advanced practice provider visits. Furthermore, the average length of stay in each also varies.

Inpatient Rehabilitation Facility

An IRF provides a level of care that is more intensive than the other forms of postacute discharge. Therefore, the patients who are recommended for this level of care need to tolerate a more rigorous therapy program. The patients who are recommended for this this level of care require a team approach that involves multiple disciplines including close physician care, skilled nursing care, rehabilitation psychology services, physical therapy, occupational therapy, speech-language therapy, recreational therapy, prosthetic/orthotic services, nutrition services, social work, and case management.

Table 1
Levels of rehabilitation care available in the United States

Level of Care	Hours/Day of Therapy	Days/Week of Therapy
Inpatient rehabilitation facility	3–5	5–7
Long-term acute hospital	1–3	3–5
Skilled nursing facility	1–3	3–5
Outpatient	1–3	1–5
Home care	1	2–3

Because the rehabilitation program is more intensive, the lengths of stay in acute rehabilitation facilities are shorter than other facilities with an average stay of approximately 12 days. The types of patient who are admitted to IRFs include stroke, fractures of the lower extremity, brain injury, spinal cord injury, amputations, debility, and other neurologic conditions (**Table 2**).

To qualify as an IRF for Medicare payment, facilities must meet the Medicare conditions of participation for acute care hospitals. They must also:

- Have a preadmission screening process to determine that each prospective patient is likely to benefit significantly from an intensive inpatient rehabilitation program;
- Ensure that the patient receives close medical supervision and provide—through qualified personnel—rehabilitation nursing, physical therapy, occupational therapy, and, as needed, speech-language pathology and psychological (including neuropsychological) services, social services, and orthotic and prosthetic services;
- Have a medical director of rehabilitation with training or experience in rehabilitation who provides services in the facility on a full-time basis for freestanding IRFs or at least 20 hours per week for hospital-based IRF units;
- Use a coordinated interdisciplinary team led by a rehabilitation physician, which includes a rehabilitation nurse, a social worker or case manager, and a licensed therapist from each therapy discipline involved in the patient's treatment;
- Have a plan of treatment of each patient who is established, reviewed, and revised as needed by a physician in consultation with other professional personnel who provide services to the patient; and

Table 2
Diagnosis treated in inpatient rehabilitation facilities

Condition	% Cases Admitted Under Medicare to IRFs in 2017
Stroke	20.5
Other neurologic conditions	15
Fracture of the lower extremity	10.4
Debility	10.6
Brain injury	10.7
Other orthopedic conditions	7.9
Cardiac conditions	5.5
Major joint replacement of lower extremity	4.4
Spinal cord injury	4.9
All other	9.8

Abbreviation: IRFs, inpatient rehabilitation facilities.

"Other neurologic conditions" includes multiple sclerosis, Parkinson disease, polyneuropathy, and neuromuscular disorders. "Fracture of the lower extremity" includes hip, pelvis, and femur fractures. Patients with debility have generalized deconditioning not attributable to other conditions. "Other orthopedic conditions" excludes fractures of the hip, pelvis, and femur, and hip and knee replacements. "All other" includes conditions such as amputations, arthritis, and pain syndrome. *Adapted from* Medicare Payment Advisory Commission (MedPAC). Inpatient rehabilitation facility services. In: Report to the congress: Medicare payment policy, March 2019:258; with permission.

- Meet the compliance threshold, which requires that no less than 60% of patients admitted to an IRF have as a primary diagnosis or comorbidity at least 1 of 13 conditions specified by the Centers for Medicare & Medicaid Services. The intent of the compliance threshold is to distinguish IRFs from acute care hospitals. If an IRF does not meet the compliance threshold, Medicare pays for all its cases on the basis of the inpatient hospital prospective payment system (PPS) rather than the IRF PPS.

The patient must have had any of the following:

- Stroke
- Spinal cord injury
- Congenital deformity
- Amputation
- Major multiple trauma
- Fracture of femur (hip fracture)
- Brain injury
- Neurologic disorders, including multiple sclerosis, motor neuron disease, polyneuropathy, muscular dystrophy, and Parkinson disease
- Burns
- Active, polyarticular rheumatoid arthritis, psoriatic arthritis, and seronegative arthropathies
- Systemic vasculidities with joint inflammation
- Severe or advanced osteoarthritis involving 2 or more major weight-bearing joints
- Knee or hip joint replacement, or both, during an acute hospitalization immediately preceding the inpatient rehabilitation stay, and also meet one or more of the following specific criteria:
  - The patient underwent bilateral knee or bilateral hip joint replacement surgery during the acute hospital admission immediately preceding the IRF admission.
  - The patient is extremely obese with a body mass index of at least 50 at the time of admission to the IRF.
  - The patient is aged 85 years or older at the time of admission to the IRF.[1]

There are also strict admission criteria for individual patients. Based on Medicare guidelines, before being admitted to an IRF program the patient must have a preadmission screening that is completed by a physician. The screening is in place to ensure that the patient being considered for admission will benefit significantly from the multidisciplinary rehabilitation program.[2] Medical necessity is established once the patient is determined to have the following characteristics:

- Require active and ongoing intervention of multiple therapy disciplines (physical therapy [PT], occupational therapy [OT], speech-language pathology [SLP], or prosthetics/orthotics), at least one of which must be PT or OT;
- Require an intensive rehabilitation therapy program, generally consisting of:
  - 3 hours of therapy per day at least 5 days per week; or
  - In certain well-documented cases, at least 15 hours of intensive rehabilitation therapy within a 7-consecutive day period, beginning with the date of admission;
- Reasonably be expected to actively participate in, and benefit significantly from, the intensive rehabilitation therapy program (the patient's condition and function status are such that the patient can reasonably be expected to make measurable improvement, expected to be made within a prescribed period of time, and as a

result of the intensive rehabilitation therapy program, that will be of practical value to improve the patient's functional capacity or adaptation to impairments);

- Require physician supervision by a rehabilitation physician, with face-to-face visits at least 3 days per week to assess the patient both medically and functionally and to modify the course of treatment as needed; and
- Require an intensive and coordinated interdisciplinary team approach to the delivery of rehabilitative care.[3]

The high intensity of IRF programs comes with a cost. In 2017, $7.9 billion in Medicare dollars were spent on about 380,000 patient admissions to IRFs.[2] IRFs are not paid under the Medicare hospital PPSs, but instead under a separate IRF PPS.[4] The current Medicare payment rates for IRF is based on a base payment rate that is, adjusted for geographic differences in the cost of labor, location of facility (rural location, teaching facilities, and facilities with a high ratio of low income patients have a higher adjustment for pay), and patient characteristics. The Medicare base payment rate for 2019 was $16,021.[5] The patient characteristics are known as "case-mix groups," and these groups are based on the reason for admission (such as amputation or stroke), age of the patient, and Functional Independence Measure (FIM). The patients in each group are further subdivided into levels based on the number of medical comorbidities.[5] However, in 2020, payment rates for Medicare are going to change. Starting in 2020, Medicare will no longer use the FIM score as a modifier to adjust payments, but will start using what is known as IRF Quality Reporting Program (QRP). The main difference between FIM and QRP is that FIM scoring system is based on the patient's lowest level of function, while QRP looks at the average function over a period of time. Even with the change in the way facilities are scoring individual patient function, the Center for Medicare Services projects that these changes will not affect overall budget toward inpatient rehabilitation admissions. However, with this change, the number of different case-mix groups will decrease.[2]

Skilled Nursing Facility

An SNF is a postacute level of care that provides skilled services to patients after an acute hospitalization. Skilled services include care that requires the expertise of a nurse and rehabilitation therapy from PT, OT, and/or SLP. The length of stay in an SNF is generally longer than in an IRF and the rehabilitation therapies are less intensive, with the average stay in an SNF being 25 days. The types of patients who are admitted to an SNF after an acute hospital stay include stroke, surgical procedures, pneumonia, heart failure, sepsis, chronic obstructive pulmonary disease, renal failure, urinary tract infections, shock, and joint replacement.[6]

To qualify for SNF level of care, Medicare guidelines stipulate that the patient be discharged from a medically necessary acute inpatient hospitalization. The admission must be for at least 3 qualifying days. The time spent in an emergency room or under observation level of care does not count toward the 3-day requirement. The patient must also be transferred to the SNF within 30 days of discharge from the qualifying 3-day hospital stay.[7] The patient must also require skilled services 7 days per week or, if their SNF admission is based only on skilled rehabilitative services, then they would need to require the services for at least 5 days per week.[7] To qualify for rehabilitative therapies at the SNF level, the patient does not need to have a potential for improvement, the patient will only need to have rehabilitative therapies that require the expertise of the skilled rehabilitative therapist.[7] This differs significantly from the expectations of patients entering the IRF level of care, where the patient is expected to improve from the therapies provided.[3]

Examples of skilled services that require nursing level of care include the administration of intravenous antibiotics and intramuscular injections, gastrostomy tube feedings, tracheostomy care, wound treatments (stage 3 or greater or widespread skin disease), monitoring of a changing medical condition, and teaching patient's how to manage their own treatments. Examples of skilled services performed by rehabilitation specialists include assessment of the patient, therapeutic exercises, gait training, range of motion, and maintenance therapy.[7–10]

In 2017, Medicare spent $28.4 billion on 2.3 million patient stays at the SNF level of care. Medicare will pay for up to 100 days of SNF care with each illness that is treated for a medically necessary 3-day hospital stay. Medicare pays 100% of the stay for the first 20 days. After day 20, patients must pay copayments for each day admitted in an SNF. In 2019, this copayment was $170.50 for each day in the SNF.[6] The PPS that is set up for SNF level of care pays the facilities on a per day basis instead of a set amount for the entire stay in the SNF. The amount paid for each day of stay in the SNF is based on which resource utilization group (RUG) the patient is in. RUGs are determined by a patient-assessment tool called the Minimum Data Set. From October 1, 2019, there is a change to how Medicare reimburses for SNF level of care.[6] Payments will no longer be based on minutes of therapy and it will be based on 5 categories of patient characteristics including nursing, rehabilitation therapies, nontherapy ancillary (such as medications), and room and board. The 5 categories are added together to establish a per day payment amount for the individual patient. The payment categories will be adjusted as the patient's needs change throughout the stay in the SNF. The Center for Medicare Services is intending that this change be a budget-neutral change; however, the payments will be redistributed from those who have the highest rehabilitation needs to those who have the highest medical care needs. This is expected to increase access to medications and complex medical care in the SNF.

Long-Term Acute Care

LTAC is a postacute level of care that is intended for medically complex patients with chronic critical illnesses who require extended acute care for their medical conditions.[11] Based on Medicare regulations, an LTAC must meet 2 conditions: (1) the facility must meet Medicare's conditions to qualify as an acute care hospital; and (2) the average length of stay for certain patients must be at least 25 days.[11] LTACs were first created as a place to send patients who were difficult to wean from the ventilator.[12,13] In 2017, more than half of the cases admitted to LTAC under Medicare were admitted for respiratory failure or mechanical ventilation. Patients admitted to LTAC include those who have had an extended length of stay in the intensive care unit. However, LTAC is also used for less acutely ill patients (**Table 3**).[11]

The cost of LTAC to Medicare was 4.5 billion for about 116,000 admissions in 2017.[11] The current Medicare payment system for LTACs uses a Medicare severity long-term care diagnosis-related group (MS-LTC-DRG). Patients are grouped into the MS-LTC-DRG by their diagnosis, procedures performed, age, sex, and discharge status. Each MS-LTC-DRG has a predetermined length of stay and thus a different pay rate. Payments for each MS-LTC-DRG are also adjusted by "short-stay outlier" LTAC stays that are shorter than average; and "High Cost Outlier" for LTAC stays that are higher than average cost.[14]

Table 3
Diagnoses treated in long-term acute care

Medicare Severity Long-Term Care Diagnosis-Related Group	% Discharges from LTAC in 2017
Pulmonary edema and respiratory failure	22.1
Respiratory system diagnosis with ventilator support 96+ h	20.8
Respiratory system diagnosis with ventilator support </ = 96 h	4.4
Septicemia without ventilator support 96+ h with major complication or comorbidity	3.8
Aftercare with complication or comorbidity/major complication or comorbidity	3.0
Other respiratory system operating room procedures with major complication or comorbidity	2.6
Renal failure with major complication or comorbidity	2.4
Tracheostomy with ventilator support 96+ h or primary diagnosis except face, mouth, and neck without major operating room procedure	2.3
Extensive operating room procedure unrelated to principal diagnosis with major complication or comorbidity	2.0
Osteomyelitis with major complication or comorbidity	1.6
Respiratory infections and inflammations with major complication or comorbidity	1.5
Skin ulcers with major complication or comorbidity	1.5
Chronic obstructive pulmonary disease with major complication or comorbidity	1.4
Postoperative and posttraumatic infections with major complication or comorbidity	1.3
Other circulatory system diagnosis with major complication or comorbidity	1.2
Complications of treatment with major complication or comorbidity	1.2
Aftercare, musculoskeletal system, and connective tissue with major complication or comorbidity	1.1
Heat failure and shock with major complication or comorbidity	1.1
Degenerative nervous system disorders with major complication or comorbidity	1.1
Major gastrointestinal disorders with peritoneal infections with major complication or comorbidity	0.8

Abbreviation: LTAC, long-term acute care.
Adapted from Medicare Payment Advisory Commission (MedPAC). Long-term care hospital services. In: Report to the congress: Medicare payment policy, March 2019:292; with permission.

Home Health Care Services

Home health care service (HHCS) is a postacute level of care provided within a patient's home. HHCS include: rehabilitation therapies, social work, intermittent nursing care, and intermittent home health aides. Home health care is intended for those patients who only need intermittent services (less than 8 hours per day).[15] The patient must also have homebound status.[16] A patient who has homebound status is allowed to leave their home to receive health care services (which also includes attending adult day care centers). Furthermore, the patient may leave their home occasionally for nonmedical activities for short periods of time. These visits can include attending religious services, trips to the barber, and attending a funeral or graduation.[16,17] There is no need for a hospital stay to qualify for home health care. A physician must have a face-to-face encounter with the patient to certify eligibility.[15]

In 2017, Medicare spent $17.7 billion on HHCS for 3.4 million patients.[15] Medicare pays for HHCS in 60-day episodes. The pay rates are based on which home health resource group (HHRG) the patient falls into. A tool called the Outcome and Assessment Information Set determines the HHRGs. The tool takes into account medical severity, functional limitations, and number of therapy visits. In 2018, base payment for a 60-day episode was $3039.64.[18] In 2020 there is going to be a change to the Medicare payment system to HHCSs. The change will adjust the 60-day episode to a 30-day episode, the number of therapy visits will be eliminated as a factor for payment, and a new categorization of patients into groups. The new categorization will be known as the Patient-Driven Groupings Model (PDGM). The PDGM will categorize groups based on episode timing, referral source, clinical category, functional/cognitive level, and presence of comorbidities.[15] The prediction is that this change to the Medicare payment system will reduce payments give to agencies that provide more therapy services and increase payments to agencies that provide more nursing services.[15]

Outcomes in Differing Levels of Rehabilitation Care

To select the appropriate level of care for a given patient, the clinician should seek to understand the outcomes in terms of patient safety, functional gains, and cost of care. There certainly exists significant overlap in the types of patients treated at each of these levels of care. Unfortunately, there exist no prospective, randomized, controlled trials of levels of care for various populations due to ethical concerns. There are some retrospective population studies looking at subgroups of patients by diagnosis, and comparing outcomes in different settings. These studies often try to control for case-mix complexity. However, they fail to account for several factors that influence outcome. These include psychosocial supports, environmental barriers at home, patient tolerance for therapy intensity, and patient motivation to participate. In addition, different tools are used to measure the degree of disability in each of these settings, making it difficult to make head-to-head comparisons among them. With these caveats, we will review the literature on comparison studies for the following diagnostic groups: stroke, elective joint replacement, and amputations.

Stroke

Several studies have concluded that patients who are admitted to IRFs have better functional outcomes compared with patients discharged to other levels of care. Chan and colleagues[19] found, in their prospective cohort study, that at 6 months, patients discharged to IRFs had statistically significantly higher functional improvements than patients who were discharged to SNFs. Similarly, in a systematic review by Alcusky and colleagues,[20] all but one of the studies found higher functional gains in stroke patients who were admitted to IRFs compared with those admitted to SNFs. This study also found that patients who were admitted to IRFs were more likely to be discharged to the community. Kane and colleagues[21] studied functional outcomes in Medicare patients at 6 weeks, which showed that patients who were discharged to IRFs also had statistically significantly higher improvements in their activities of daily living dependency scores when compared with those discharged to SNFs.

Rehospitalization is another area of important outcome. In the prospective cohort study by Chan and colleagues, it was found that the rehospitalization rates over the

6-month period of the study were similar for all the patients discharged to IRFs, SNFs, home health care, and outpatient services. Kane and colleagues[21] found that the rehospitalization rates at 1 year after discharge from SNFs was 22%, while those for IRFs were greater than 25%. The same study found that rehospitalization rate at 1 year to patients discharged to HHCS was the lowest at 20%. However, a different study found opposite findings and determined that patients who were admitted to IRFs were less likely to be rehospitalized than patients admitted to SNFs in other studies.[20] Kind and colleagues[22] found lower readmission rates from IRFs than SNFs across all racial groups. Middleton and colleagues[23–26] looked at readmission rates at 30 and 90 days for IRFs versus SNFs in ischemic and hemorrhagic stroke. In ischemic stroke, 10.2% of IRF patients were readmitted at 30 days and 21.4% at 90 days, whereas for SNF patients those numbers were 11.5% and 23.8%. Similarly in hemorrhagic stroke IRF patients were also readmitted at a significantly lower rate.

Kane and colleagues[21] analyzed mortality rate as one of their outcomes. They found that patients admitted to IRFs had lower rates of mortality than patients admitted to SNFs at 6 weeks, 6 months, and 1 year after stroke ($P<.01$). Similarly, Buntin and colleagues[27] and Kind and colleagues also found significantly lower mortality rates among stroke patients discharged from acute care to IRFs as opposed to SNFs.

Amputation

The studies that have analyzed outcomes after amputation in relation to postacute level of care have seemed to agree that patients had better overall outcomes when admitted to IRFs after acute amputation. A study by Dillingham and Pezzin[28] found that patients who were admitted to IRFs for rehabilitation had a significantly higher survival rate and were less likely to experience reamputation. They also found that patients who were admitted to SNFs had better outcomes in regard to mortality and likelihood of receiving a prosthesis when compared with patients who were discharged directly home. The same study found that patients admitted to IRFs were less likely to be readmitted to acute care in the year following their amputation. A different study by Vogel and colleagues[29] looked at all risk factors associated with 30-day readmission after lower extremity amputation in patients with vascular disease. The study found that patients who were at the highest risk for readmission included those with hypertension, heart failure, administration of antihistamines, surgery at a teaching hospital, urgent or emergent admission, below the knee amputation, discharge disposition to an SNF, or complications including surgical site infection. A study by Curran and colleagues[30,31] also found that readmission was higher in patients with chronic nursing home residency, nonelective surgery, nonhome discharge, preoperative congestive heart failure, preoperative dialysis, and previous revascularization or amputation.

Joint Replacement

A study known as Joints I was a prospective observational cohort study by DeJong and colleagues[32–34] that compared outcomes between both IRFs and SNFs in patients with nontraumatic joint replacement. They found that the volume of patients with joint replacements that a facility admitted per year was important to outcomes. They found that both IRFs and SNFs that had medium volume had better outcomes. However, the Joints II study found no differences in the long-term outcomes between the facilities. The study analyzed outcomes at 7.5 months after admission to rehabilitation after joint replacement.

SUMMARY

In the United States, we are blessed with many options for postacute care: IRFs, LTACH, SNFs, HHAs, and OP. However, choosing the appropriate level of care can be a daunting task. It requires interdisciplinary input and involvement of all stakeholders. The decision should be informed by outcomes data specific to the patient's diagnosis, impairments, and psychosocial supports.

DISCLOSURE

The authors have nothing to disclose.

REFERENCES

1. Center for Medicare Services. Fact sheet #1 inpatient rehabilitation facility classification requirements 2005. Available at: https://www.cms.gov/Medicare/Medicare-Fee-for-Service-Payment/InpatientRehabFacPPS/downloads/fs1class req.pdf. Accessed May 17, 2019.

2. Medicare Payment Advisory Commission (MedPAC). Chapter 10: Inpatient rehabilitation facility services. In: Report to the congress: Medicare payment policy Washington, DC: March 2019. p. 249–77.

3. Department of Health and Human Services. Centers for Medicare and Medicaid Services. Inpatient rehabilitation therapy services: complying with documentation requirements. Medicare Learning Network Web site. 2012. Available at: https://www.cms.gov/Outreach-and-Education/Medicare-Learning-Network-MLN/MLN Products/downloads/Inpatient_Rehab_Fact_Sheet_ICN905643.pdf. Accessed May 17, 2019.

4. Centers for Medicare & Medicaid Services. Inpatient rehabilitation facilities. CMS.gov: Centers for Medicare & Medicaid Services Web site. 2012. Available at: https://www.cms.gov/Medicare/Provider-Enrollment-and-Certification/Certifica tionandComplianc/InpatientRehab.html. Accessed May 18, 2019.

5. Medicare Payment Advisory Commission (MedPAC). Inpatient rehabilitation facilities payment system. paymentbasics Web site. 2018. Available at: http://www.medpac.gov/docs/default-source/payment-basics/medpac_payment_basics_18_irf_final_sec.pdf?sfvrsn=0. Accessed May 17, 2019.

6. Medicare Payment Advisory Commission (MedPAC). Chapter 8: Skilled nursing facility services. In: Report to the congress: Medicare Payment Policy. Washington, DC: March 2019. p. 191–224.

7. Chapter 8 - coverage of extended care (SNF) services under hospital insurance. Medicare Benefit Policy Manual Web site. 2018. Available at: https://www.cms.gov/Regulations-and-Guidance/Guidance/Manuals/downloads/bp10 2c08.pdf. Accessed May 19, 2019.

8. Center for Medicare Services. Nursing home/skilled nursing facility care. Washington, DC: Center For Medicare Advocacy Web site; 2019. Available at: https://www.medicareadvocacy.org/medicare-info/skilled-nursing-facility-snf-services/#whats covered. Accessed 05, 2019.

9. Brown JG. Nursing home resident assessment: resource utilization groups. Washington, DC: Department of Health and Human Services: Office of Inspector General Web site; 2001. Available at: https://oig.hhs.gov/oei/reports/oei-02-99-00041.pdf. Accessed May 19, 2019.

10. Minimum data set (MDS) - version 3.0. . 2011. Available at: https://www.cms.gov/Research-Statistics-Data-and-Systems/Computer-Data-and-Systems/Minimum-Data-Set-3-0-Public-Reports/index.

11. Medicare Payment Advisory Commission (MedPAC). Chapter 11: Long-term care hospital services. In: Report to the congress: Medicare payment policy. Washington, DC: March 2019. p. 279–307.

12. Eskildsen MA. Long-term acute care: a review of the literature. J Am Geriatr Soc 2007;55(5):775–9.

13. Makam AN, Nguyen OK, Xuan L, et al. Long-term acute care hospital use of non-mechanically ventilated hospitalized older adults. J Am Geriatr Soc 2018;66(11):2112–9.

14. Center for Medicare Services. Long-term care hospital prospective payment system. mln booklet Web site. 2018. Available at: https://www.cms.gov/Outreach-and-Education/Medicare-Learning-Network-MLN/MLNProducts/Downloads/Long-Term-Care-Hospital-PPS-Fact-Sheet-ICN006956.pdf. Accessed May 28, 2019.

15. Medicare Payment Advisory Commission (MedPAC). Chapter 9: Home health care services. In: Report to the congress: Medicare Payment Policy. Washington, DC: March 2019. p. 225–48.

16. Center for Medicare Services. Chapter 7—home health services. Medicare benefit policy manual web site. Available at: https://www.cms.gov/Regulations-and-Guidance/Guidance/Manuals/downloads/bp102c07.pdf. Accessed June 02, 2019.

17. Loeffler H, Simpson C, Center for Medicare Services. Certifying patients for the Medicare home health benefit. MLN Connects: National Provider Call Web site 2015. Available at: https://www.cms.gov/Outreach-and-Education/Outreach/NPC/Downloads/2014-12-16-HHBenefit-HL.pdf. Accessed June 02, 2019.

18. Medicare Payment Advisory Commission (MedPAC). Home health care services payment system. Payment Basics Web site. 2018. Available at: http://www.medpac.gov/docs/default-source/payment-basics/medpac_payment_basics_18_hha_final_sec.pdf?sfvrsn=0. Accessed June 02, 2019.

19. Chan L, Elizabeth Sandel M, Jette AM, et al. Does postacute care site matter? A longitudinal study assessing functional recovery after a stroke. Arch Phys Med Rehabil 2012;94(4):622–9.

20. Alcusky M, Ulbricht CM, Lapane KL. Postacute care setting, facility characteristics, and poststroke outcomes: a systematic review. Arch Phys Med Rehabil 2018;99(6):1124–40.e9.

21. Kane RL, Chen Q, Finch M, et al. Functional outcomes of posthospital care for stroke and hip fracture patients under medicare. J Am Geriatr Soc 1998;46(12):1525–33.

22. Kind AJ, Smith MA, Liou J, et al. Discharge destination's effect on bounce-back risk in black, white, and hispanic acute ischemic stroke patients. Arch Phys Med Rehabil 2010;91:189–95.

23. Middleton A, Kuo YF, Graham JE, et al. Readmission patterns over 90-day episodes of care among medicare fee-for-service beneficiaries discharged to post-acute care. J Am Med Dir Assoc 2018;19(10):896–901.

24. Ottenbacher KJ, Smith PM, Illig SB, et al. Characteristics of persons rehospitalized after stroke rehabilitation. Arch Phys Med Rehabil 2001;82(10):1367–74.

25. Chung DM, Niewczyk P, Divita M, et al. Predictors of discharge to acute care after inpatient rehabilitation in severely affected stroke patients. Am J Phys Med Rehabil 2012;91(5):387–92.

26. Kushner DS, Johnson-Greene D. Association of urinary incontinence with cognition, transfers and discharge destination in acute stroke inpatient rehabilitation. J Stroke Cerebrovasc Dis 2018;27(10):2677–82.

27. Buntin MB, Colla CH, Deb P, et al. Medicare spending and outcomes after postacute care for stroke and hip fracture. Med Care 2010;48:776–84.

28. Dillingham TR, Pezzin LE. Rehabilitation setting and associated mortality and medical stability among persons with amputations. Arch Phys Med Rehabil 2008;89(6):1038–45. Available at: https://doi-org.proxy1.library.jhu.edu/10.1016/j.apmr.2007.11.034.

29. Vogel TR, Smith JB, Kruse RL. Risk factors for thirty-day readmissions after lower extremity amputation in patients with vascular disease. PM R 2018;10(12):1321–9.

30. Curran T, Zhang JQ, Lo RC, et al. Risk factors and indications for readmission after lower extremity amputation in the American College of Surgeons national surgical quality improvement program. J Vasc Surg 2014;60(5):1315–24.

31. Ries Z, Rungprai C, Harpole B, et al. Incidence, risk factors, and causes for thirty-day unplanned readmissions following primary lower-extremity amputation in patients with diabetes. J Bone Joint Surg Am 2015;97(21):1774–80.

32. Dejong G, Horn SD, Smout RJ, et al. Joint replacement rehabilitation outcomes on discharge from skilled nursing facilities and inpatient rehabilitation facilities. Arch Phys Med Rehabil 2009;90(8):1284–96.

33. DeJong G, Tian W, Smout RJ, et al. Long-term outcomes of joint replacement rehabilitation patients discharged from skilled nursing and inpatient rehabilitation facilities. Arch Phys Med Rehabil 2009;90(8):1306–16.

34. Falvey JR, Bade MJ, Forster JE, et al. Home-health-care physical therapy improves early functional recovery of Medicare beneficiaries after total knee arthroplasty. J Bone Joint Surg Am 2018;100(20):1728–34.

Moving?

Make sure your subscription moves with you!

To notify us of your new address, find your **Clinics Account Number** (located on your mailing label above your name), and contact customer service at:

Email: journalscustomerservice-usa@elsevier.com

800-654-2452 (subscribers in the U.S. & Canada)
314-447-8871 (subscribers outside of the U.S. & Canada)

Fax number: 314-447-8029

Elsevier Health Sciences Division
Subscription Customer Service
3251 Riverport Lane
Maryland Heights, MO 63043

*To ensure uninterrupted delivery of your subscription, please notify us at least 4 weeks in advance of move.

Printed and bound by CPI Group (UK) Ltd, Croydon, CR0 4YY

03/10/2024

01040408-0016